A Nurse's Story

LOUISE CURTIS

WITH SARAH JOHNSON

PAN BOOKS

First published 2020 by Pan Books
an imprint of Pan Macmillan
The Smithson, 6 Briset Street, London EC1M 5NR
Associated companies throughout the world
www.panmacmillan.com

ISBN 978-1-5290-5893-2

1 3 5 7 9 8 6 4 2

A CIP catalogue record for this book is available from the British Library.

Typeset by Palimpsest Book Production Limited, Falkirk, Stirlingshire
Printed and bound by CPI Group (UK) Ltd, Croydon, CR0 4YY

Visit www.panmacmillan.com to read more about all our books
and to buy them. You will also find features, author interviews and
news of any author events, and you can sign up for e-newsletters
so that you're always first to hear about our new releases.

Louise Curtis is an advanced clinical practitioner at an A&E in a major trauma centre. She is a nurse by background and has been working in the emergency department for eight years, both as a staff nurse and deputy sister. She has volunteered abroad in South Africa, Thailand, Uganda and Ethiopia, caring for disabled orphans, and HIV and trauma patients.

Sarah Johnson has been a journalist for twelve years, seven of them at the *Guardian*. She founded and edits the Blood, Sweat and Tears series, which features first-person accounts of working in and receiving healthcare. As a writer, she specializes in mental health and other aspects of healthcare in the UK and abroad.

To our parents, and to those
who suffer whose voices go unheard

Authors' note

The stories told here are all grounded in reality, but we have changed names of patients (if mentioned) and identifying details so that no one can be recognized. Many of the individual patients described are typical of a large number of A&E attendees.

Occasionally, a story may draw upon a composite of different experiences from Louise's career, to ensure patient confidentiality is upheld.

Louise Curtis is a pseudonym.

Prologue

A woman in her forties lay before me. She was struggling to breathe, she looked exhausted and her oxygen levels were dangerously low. Fifteen minutes ago, she had been fine. Now, it was time for intensive care to get involved and for her to go on a ventilator. I knew that her chances of survival were growing less with each passing moment. I'd heard about the rapid deterioration in coronavirus patients, but this was the first time it had played out in front of me. I couldn't help feeling responsible. Had I somehow brought about this series of events? The guilt was overwhelming.

Shirley had been admitted into A&E about fifty minutes before I came on shift. The doctor who I had taken over from had ordered some blood tests and we were waiting for a chest X-ray. She had also been tested for Covid-19 but we didn't yet know the result. When I met her, she was very worried; I wasn't.

'Am I going to be OK?' she asked me.

'You'll be fine, you just need a bit of oxygen,' I replied. At the time, I honestly believed it.

I looked at her notes. She'd had nine days of coronavirus symptoms, but none were terribly serious. She had no prior medical history, was fit and healthy and not part of the high-risk group who were more susceptible to succumbing to the virus. I couldn't understand why she was so anxious.

Some years back when I was newly qualified as a nurse, there was a man in his thirties who came in with chest pain. He was normally fit and healthy and looked fine. He was due to go to a ward elsewhere in the hospital to wait for a blood test to come back.

'Am I going to be OK?' he said.

'Of course,' I replied.

'Will you tell my wife I love her and tell her to look after the baby.'

I reiterated that he would be fine, but passed the message on when his wife called up to check on him. She said she'd be arriving soon. I later found out that a few hours after he had gone up to the ward, he had a cardiac arrest and died. Ever since, I've had this gut feeling, a sense of dread in the pit of my stomach, when patients think they're going to die. Lots of healthcare professionals talk about it, and it's usually a warning sign. I did not get that feeling with Shirley, however. And knowing that makes it even worse. I even reassured her mother that everything looked as though it would be all right. I could tell she was also really worried on the phone.

'She's not going to end up in intensive care, is she?' she asked.

'We would discharge her home if only she didn't need a bit of oxygen to top her up,' I said reassuringly. 'She's going to be fine. I don't anticipate that she will need to go into the intensive care unit.'

That was the only time I spoke to her. I never got a chance to phone her mother back and speak to her myself. The ward would do it, but it should have been me to break the news.

Back on the isolation unit, Shirley kept ringing her bell. I had spent a long time with her explaining everything as clearly as I could. A short while later, one of the nurses asked me to explain again because Shirley had said she didn't know what was happening. Was she just a worrier or was she starting to become seriously unwell? I checked her over again and she seemed fine. Her observations – oxygen saturation, heart rate, temperature, etc. – didn't look bad.

Then we got her chest X-ray back and it was the worst one I had ever seen. Her entire left lung was infiltrated with Covid-19. There was very little air getting in there. One of the consultants in another area of A&E rang to check I'd seen it. 'I'm looking at it now,' I said. He told me to call up the respiratory ward. I did and we agreed that Shirley would go there.

There was only one crew that could transport Covid-positive patients and so we had about a two-hour wait before they arrived. It was often the same two crew members, so I assumed that the others were shielding because they had health problems and were high risk. Either that, or the funding wasn't there. In the meantime I went in regularly to check up on Shirley, who was still very worried. Her bag of fluids finished. 'Do I need another one?' she asked desperately. I prescribed her a second bag. Her blood pressure was teetering on the low side, her heart rate was up and her sodium was a little low too. All three things could be helped by some fluids.

When the transport arrived, a nurse went in to check on Shirley. It's policy to check a patient's observations before they go anywhere. The nurse came back. 'Shirley's oxygen level is low and it's fallen rapidly. I think you need to come and see her,' she said.

I went in to check. She was slumped halfway down the trolley, which was not unusual – they must be slippy as it happens all the time – but she was alert and had colour in her cheeks. We got her into a better position, expecting her oxygen levels to rise now that she was sat upright, but as I stood there and watched, they didn't get any better. The crew could not transport her and everyone was frustrated because a bed had been made ready, but I maintained she wasn't fit to be moved.

A little while later I took an arterial blood sample to check her oxygen levels. They were very low. I went to my senior in resuscitation and told him I was worried.

'Bring her here into resus,' he said. 'We'll give her some more oxygen.'

We gave her the maximum but nothing was helping. I got on the phone to intensive care.

A doctor from the ICU came down, decided she needed to be intubated and took her away. By this time it was beyond my shift finish and I was meant to have gone home. I felt I couldn't leave, though. I wanted to know that she was going to be OK. The registrar came over as it was time for me to leave.

'Right, Louise, can you tell me what happened with this patient?'

'It all happened so quickly. She was fine and then suddenly she wasn't.'

'What drugs did you prescribe her?'

I told him everything I'd done before he rushed off to see another patient. He offered me no reassurance and that conversation, and all that preceded it, left me feeling horrendous. Not only had I potentially misled her mother, but I wondered if my actions had somehow contributed towards Shirley's deterioration. 'This is all my fault,' I thought. I was reminded of how little I felt I knew and it was a stark reminder of the fragility of life and that, despite all my training, sometimes I feel I don't really know what I'm doing.

It was the end of my shift and I was getting undressed in the changing room when a colleague came in who had admitted Shirley when she first came in to A&E.

'How is she doing?' she asked.

'She's gone to intensive care,' I said.

'Yeah, I knew something bad was on its way,' she replied.

Just before I left to go home, I went into the office and saw my colleague Phoebe sitting at the computer doing some work. She was in the same role as me but had a few more years' experience.

'Hey Louise, how's your shift been?'

'I feel terrible, Phoebe,' I replied.

'Why? What happened? Let's talk it over.'

I told her about what had happened with Shirley and that she was now in intensive care fighting for her life.

'I'm so scared I did something wrong. What if she dies and it's all my fault?'

'Oh my goodness, stop! You did the best you could and it sounds like you didn't do anything wrong at all. Covid-19 is a new virus. No one knows exactly what they're doing and if they say they do, they're lying. The research around what to prescribe for patients is constantly changing.'

'I just feel I've got imposter syndrome and that I'm not good enough to be doing this job.'

'I can assure you that everyone gets waves of imposter syndrome at points in their career, even the most senior consultants. I get it all the time. You need to try and work through it and remember that patients are lucky to have you treating them, because you're great at your job.'

'Thanks, Phoebe, that's really kind of you to say.'

'Well, it's true. Now get off home, it's way past your finish time.'

Phoebe had made me feel better but, even so, that shift had shaken me to the core.

1

Becoming a Nurse

I am an advanced clinical practitioner (ACP) in A&E. When the coronavirus crisis took hold of the UK in March 2020, I'd been in the job for five months. I had worked as a nurse for eight years but, after three years of training, this new role saw me performing the job of a junior doctor for the first time. I'm definitely not a doctor because I didn't go through medical school. ACPs can be nurses, physiotherapists, pharmacists, paramedics or occupational therapists by background, and can end up working at the same level as a middle-grade doctor. It's a new and little-understood role in the NHS but we see patients, diagnose them and prescribe treatment. It's a lot more responsibility than what I was used to and my actions and decisions can decide whether someone lives or dies.

I was still getting used to this daunting realization and just starting to feel a bit more settled in the role when the whole world changed, almost overnight it seemed. Life and everything around me suddenly started going at breakneck speed and I, along with everyone else working in healthcare, was running to catch up, both metaphorically and literally.

But first, let me take you back to where this particular journey began for me. It's probably not where you would expect. I was determined to be the first female bishop in the UK when I left school to study theology at university. I had dreams of shaking up the male hierarchy in the church. But then, in my second year as a student, at the age of nineteen, I had a cycling accident that changed my perspective on what I wanted to do with my life.

I had decided to raise money for charity by cycling from Leeds to Paris. My best friend signed up with me and I thought it would be fun and worthwhile. As it was quite a long way, we did various training rides to build our stamina and endurance. One Sunday afternoon, I was pedalling along a country road in the Yorkshire countryside with the wind blowing in my face and my thoughts drifting off to I don't know where, when I rode over a pothole. The jolt sent me flying over the handlebars. I remember thinking, 'Oh no!' mid-flight, before I crash-landed face first on the road.

Next thing I knew I was in the back of the ambulance; my best friend, who I've known since I was three years old, was with me but was so shocked she couldn't remember my name, and the paramedics were making jokes about me ruining their morning cup of tea. They had dropped my teeth – the ones that had fallen out and that had been picked up off the road – in their stash of milk.

I arrived at the hospital. My head was taped down and all I could see was the ceiling. It was a very disturbing experience. I couldn't look around me, and I could just hear all these voices shouting things before the pain took over and I blacked out.

My memories of that stay in hospital are grim. I was on a cocktail of painkillers that I now refuse to prescribe to anyone because they're so awful. The only meaningful interaction I had with any of the staff was when the doctor asked me if I'd looked in the mirror yet. I said, 'No.' He said, 'Good. Probably best not to.'

I stayed on a ward with mostly elderly patients for five days. I had broken both my elbows so moving wasn't really much of an option. No one working on the ward took any notice of me. I can understand why now: I didn't require much care because I was young and fit, so I was left. They brought me food, but because I'd broken my elbows I couldn't lift it to my mouth so I didn't eat. I would sit there, in a drugged-up state, vomiting because of the painkillers. I had sick all down my front but with no call bell I couldn't tell anybody.

Then one day, they needed my bed so I was told to go. I was left in a hard chair by the hospital entrance while I waited for my parents to pick me up. Back at home I could hardly walk up the stairs. The pain was unbearable and I was left with a conviction that my stay in hospital had not been a good experience and that that was wrong. Surely care was meant to be better?

My memories of that time are foggy at best, but I remember my mother having to toilet me and wash me. She ran me a bath one night and put bubble bath in, which was so thoughtful and caring of her. The only thing was it was very oily so when it came to me trying to get out of the bath, I kept slipping. I couldn't use my arms to lever myself up because they were broken and Mum couldn't lift me either. I'm tall, like my father, and outgrew her in my early teens. I was so annoyed at her for using an oil-based bubble bath, and the whole experience was so embarrassing and painful. It didn't take long to see the funny side though, and I started half crying, half laughing as my legs kept giving way beneath me as soapy water lapped around me. I eventually managed to get them underneath my body and carefully stood up out of the water and onto dry land. Now when I think about it, it's really quite comical.

One thing that sticks clearly in my mind was one night when I woke up crying. I was so uncomfortable and my bed sheets were in a mess. I must have been making a lot of noise because my sister, who prides herself on her ability to sleep through almost anything, came in asking, 'Are you OK?' I wailed, 'Everything hurts and I can't get to sleep.' She straightened up my sheets and I got back in and fell asleep within minutes.

That gesture really surprised me. It made me realize what had been lacking at the hospital. If my sister could do this, then why couldn't professional nurses? I resolved to change things. I didn't want other people to go through what I had experienced; I wanted better. So I applied to study nursing after I finished my degree in theology.

I was also a big fan of *Grey's Anatomy* and thought I might meet my future 'McDreamy' husband at work. On that count, I was wrong. Although when I met my now husband Ed at university he *was* volunteering with St John Ambulance. He used to be on duty at gigs in the students' union. I remember thinking 'phwoar' and that he was really cool because he got involved if anything medical kicked off and he got gig tickets for free (a very attractive bonus when I was living on a student budget).

When we were first introduced by a mutual friend I had to leave the room because I was so shy and embarrassed. 'I've got something in my eye,' I mumbled, and made a quick exit. Luckily we met again at a fancy dress party. I'd gone as a Christmas present, I remember, and with a couple of drinks inside me for Dutch courage I managed to actually talk to him this time when he came over.

At university I spent two summers volunteering in Uganda and one working in an orphanage in Thailand. I also did a few short placements abroad – one in Uganda and one in Ethiopia – when I was training as a nurse. I had a relatively privileged upbringing and I don't think I had really been exposed to any of the suffering and inequality that I saw on those trips. Since working in A&E, however, I've realized that even though the UK has one of the strongest economies in the world, that doesn't mean there isn't poverty, and people living in dire situations. It's perhaps a bit more hidden, but I definitely see it in the emergency department.

I've always had a desire to help people; my mum told me she always thought I would go into a caring profession. It would have been helpful if she'd said this to me before I embarked on a three-year degree in theology, but never mind.

Spending some of my childhood growing up in the Sultanate of Oman also instilled in me and my sister a strong desire to see more of the world and to experience it in ways different to just passing through on holiday.

When I got into nursing, I worked for some weeks in an HIV clinic in Uganda, which involved going out to remote rural areas to do community visits. I saw a cancer patient who had HIV as well. He was emaciated, covered in flies, with pressure sores on his hips, shoulders, elbows and the back of his head. The skin had broken down so much that his bones were visible. There was a black market for drugs; vulnerable people were given anti-psychotics instead of anti-malarials and then died from malaria. I saw evidence of witchcraft; people would wear shells in the belief that they had healing powers. It was really upsetting, but it was their normal cultural practice.

I qualified as a nurse in 2012 and started work in A&E in the same hospital I'm in today. I loved the job but I also wanted to work abroad and started to research organizations that would allow me to do this. Many cited a tropical nursing diploma as a desirable qualification so I applied to the Liverpool School of Tropical Medicine. I ended up taking three weeks of my annual leave to go and live in Liverpool to do the course.

A friend had kindly said I could stay in the flat that belonged to his grandmother, who had passed away. His family are ordained in the church and so the flat contained the odd crucifix and piece of religious memorabilia. By this point, religion and I were not getting along. I struggle to believe there's a god after some of what I've seen. It was in winter, so very dark and cold. I couldn't figure out how to use the hot water, either. But I was there to study, and so I didn't mind.

The course was intense; the volume of information I had to take in was overwhelming. The tutors were awe-inspiring. I really looked up to them because their life experience was incredible. They were a bit like gods for me and I wanted to be like them. I hoped that one day I would be able to be on equal terms with them and they might acknowledge me. I was young at the time and most of the other people on the course were older and had more experience than I did. It seemed everybody had worked in Mali; it became a bit of a joke to me, to be honest. Some of the attendees were really cocky and kept going on about how many deployments they'd done. Nevertheless, hearing accounts of working in some of the major global relief efforts was humbling.

We learnt how to work in disaster zones, about common diseases and how to identify, treat and manage them. I remember looking at lots of poo samples under a microscope. That was a bit unnerving – I had had tropical diseases and my poo would have been sent off to be examined and then perhaps used as a sample to help teach others like me doing the course.

After one trip to Uganda, I tested positive for bilharzia, a type of parasitic worm infection carried by freshwater snails. I had been swimming in a lake and knew I should get tested for it six weeks after I got back. I didn't have any symptoms but was told I had it quite badly; the danger is that you can be asymptomatic and then suddenly go into multiple organ failure and die. Ed's first question was, 'Is it contagious?' How loving.

Another highlight from the course was watching a man milking a snake's glands so that it produced its venom, which could then be used to create an anti-venom. It was really odd to watch; there was a man holding a snake by its head with one hand while the other was moving up and down in what I can only describe as a masturbatory motion. All the while, I was stood right next to it, feeling very uncomfortable and wishing I could be back looking at poo samples. The whole room was full of snakes. I hate snakes. There were also boxes containing huge spiders that looked like they were being electrocuted inside because they were jumping erratically all over the place.

Never did I think then that the UK would come to be one of the worst-hit countries in the world at a time when a new virus was sweeping over the planet. After all that training and dreaming of going to another country to help, a global health emergency ended up coming to me.

In August 2018 Ed and I got married in a woodland ceremony in North Yorkshire, near to where I grew up and where my parents still lived.

My eighty-five-year-old father walked me down the aisle in a bright yellow sunflower waistcoat, jazzy tie and a top hat. Looking back, I didn't realize at the time how precious the memory of that moment, as I linked my arm in his, would become to me. Dad obviously hadn't got the message about not upstaging the bride but I didn't mind. My sister and I learnt from an early age that he was a colourful, head-turning, unstoppable character. You knew when he walked into a room. 'You never get a second chance to make a first impression,' he used to tell us.

My husband didn't pursue a career in healthcare; he

works in engineering. I still don't really understand what he does, and it's part funny, part awkward when my family asks him every time they see him to explain his job.

That's the thing about working in A&E: people can imagine to a certain extent what my job involves. In the emergency department, I see and experience everything in extremes. We treat everyone from the guy that sleeps rough in a shop doorway to multi-millionaire local sports stars and businessmen. When patients come through our doors, they are at their most vulnerable. It's more than that, though. In A&E we are there when people are going through perhaps the worst experience of their life. We deal in emergencies and we do it well, but it's gruesome and we can't always save everyone.

There are countless patients I'll never forget. And their stories are what eventually led to me losing my faith. The worst seem to take place at Christmas, which makes them even more tragic. One Christmas Eve in particular always sticks in my mind. I was working in resuscitation – the bit of the department where all the most critical patients come for life-saving treatment. Before they arrive, we often get a call telling us what to expect. On this occasion we knew it was a man in his thirties who had been involved in a road traffic collision.

The scene when a patient arrives is not one of chaos. Everything is silent – nobody talks – with only the bleep of machines and whatever noise other patients might be making in the background. Various professionals swoop down on us from around the hospital: the anaesthetist with an operating department practitioner in tow, the orthopaedics doctor who will assess any broken bones, the surgeon who's there for any ruptured blood vessels or abdominal bleeding, among others.

The paramedics brought this man in quickly and told us what had happened. He had just returned from an army tour in Afghanistan and had been met at the airport by his wife and newborn baby. They were driving home together when they had a head-on collision with a lorry. The wife was killed instantly, but the baby and our patient had been brought in.

He had a blood pressure and a heart rate, indicating that he was stable for now, but we were yet to discover the extent of his injuries. He did not look good. As the nurse, I was responsible with another clinician for doing the initial assessment. I looked him over from head to toe documenting what there was to try and fix. I put an oxygen saturations probe on the patient's finger, a blood pressure cuff around his arm, heart rate monitoring leads on his chest. I cut his clothes off and inserted a cannula while everyone else also got to work.

His heart soon stopped beating and he went into cardiac arrest. The trauma team – made up of senior A&E doctors – ended up cutting his chest open to try and give his heart manual massage with their hands and to stop the bleeding. But it was futile, and he died. I remember thinking: 'This is shit.'

A&E is a fast-paced environment so there was no time to stop. I had to push my feelings into a box and close the lid so I could go and see the next patient. Sometimes, they can hear what's going on and they ask me if someone has just died. I often tell them yes because what else can I say?

We also see a lot of people with mental health problems in A&E, which sometimes leaves me feeling utterly powerless. Many are young, my age (I'm now thirty-two) or younger. One case that hit me the hardest, however, was an elderly woman who had attempted suicide. She had overdosed but then woken up hours later distressed and confused. She called 999, but remembered while on the phone why she was in this state and what her intentions had been, and hung up.

Before the paramedics got to her, she had stabbed herself multiple times to the chest and abdomen with a letter-opener.

When a patient attends A&E with a mental health problem one of our first priorities is to discover what level of risk they pose to both themselves and others. We have to ask honestly and somewhat intrusively, 'What did you hope to happen when you took action to end your life?' or 'What are your plans if we send you home?' The responses range from, 'I need to feed my cats and I have work in the morning,' to 'I don't want to live any longer.' By asking these questions, we can decide what measures are needed to keep everyone safe.

When I spoke to my elderly patient, she told me, 'I don't want to be here anymore. I can't take it any longer.'

'What do you mean by "it"? Is something going on? Can you tell me about it?' I asked.

'My neighbour keeps sexually assaulting me. I'm all alone with nobody to help me. My husband died some years back and we never had children. I'm terrified every time I have to leave the house in case my neighbour's there. I only go out if I absolutely have to.'

At that point we were interrupted because the porter arrived to take her off to theatre where a surgical team would try and repair the damage to her liver and spleen. I called the hospital's safeguarding team who would follow up and determine if she was safe enough to be discharged back to her own home, or if temporary new accommodation needed to be found. I never heard anything more.

I see patients at their lowest ebb and often I don't know what happens to them. I don't get closure so am left walking around with what feels to me like a massive open wound. You have to carry on like you're absolutely fine and like nothing's happened. What is there to do? The next patient needs antibiotics. Right, on it.

It's horrible and one of the worst things about the job.

Most of the time, I'm somehow able to keep going. I have cried on a few occasions at work, but not many, and only once did my eyes well up in front of a relative. The situations that really get to me are where patients come in and there's nobody there, so I sit holding their hand while they die. This has happened on more occasions than I can remember. I don't like anyone to be alone at such a difficult time so I stay with them as long as I can. They're often unconscious so I don't know if they can hear me but I tell them, 'It's OK. You can go now.' I do it because that's what I'd want for my relative.

Another one of my worst experiences was when an elderly couple came into the department. They'd been married for sixty years and the wife had suddenly collapsed at the supper table. She'd had a spontaneous bleed on the brain. We intubated her to maintain her airway so she could keep breathing but the head scan showed she wouldn't survive.

The plan was to take the tubes out to let her pass away. In this situation, however, you don't know how quick it will be. It can take minutes, hours, or sometimes days. Telling the family this is horrendous and I hate it.

I went into the visitors' room where the husband was waiting and told him the news. He looked broken.

'What am I going to do now?' he asked me. 'She's all I've got.'

The thought of him having to go home alone was too much to bear. They didn't have any children. What could I do for him? Not a lot.

His wife ended up dying within the hour and that was it. I said goodbye to him as he said he wanted to go home. It felt callous and unfeeling, and like I, or someone, should be doing something to help him. I wished there was provision for us to do more, but we're A&E. We don't have the capacity. I'm still moved when I think about that man years later.

There are moments of joy too, however. I guess it's those that offset some of the misery and heartbreak I experience on a weekly basis. Back when I was nursing there was a girl in her late teens who came in with stomach pain. I was triaging patients that day, being the first point of contact who then decided what course of action to take for each person. I asked her to describe the pain: 'How long has it been going on and how long does it last before it goes away? Is it constant, or coming and going?'

'It's constant, but every now and then it gets a lot worse,' she told me.

'When was your last period?'

'I'm not sure.'

'Could you be pregnant?' I asked.

'No, I don't think so,' she replied.

Then, as if right on cue, a puddle of liquid appeared on the floor. Her waters had broken. I quickly took her into resus as tears streamed down her face.

'Please don't tell my dad,' she pleaded. 'He can't find out, or see me.'

An image of a brutish and violent father was building in my mind. I was getting really worried. Was it a safeguarding concern? 'Oh God,' I then thought. 'How am I going to get the mum here on her own?' The girl wanted her mother with her, but the pair were in the hospital together and knew their daughter was here. The logistics of the situation were unbelievably tricky to navigate. The team and I were so stressed. We thought we'd have to get the security team down and that it was all going to kick off and be thoroughly unpleasant for all sides.

Before we had time to plot our next steps, the dad came rushing through with his wife. The doors to resus are really flimsy and you can't lock them, so there was no keeping him out. We had not managed to get control of the situation. He entered the cubicle where his daughter was and started crying. He hugged and kissed her, and told her how proud he was of her. This was not what any of us had envisaged. On seeing the love he felt for his daughter, the whole team also started crying. We had been so anxious and scared that he was going to be awful but he turned out to be one of the loveliest people I've ever come across. She delivered a healthy baby and went home happy with her parents.

It's situations like these that have taught me to always expect the unexpected in A&E. People surprise you and catch you out.

I was once undressing a patient so I could assess him. He was quite unkempt but very well educated and was reciting poetry to me. I took one sock off, and then went to remove the other. As I took it off, one of his toes popped out. It fell, I went to catch it, juggled it in mid-air and finally grasped it before it fell on the floor. It was black all over. The patient was lying down so didn't see any of this. He was blissfully unaware. I was not. 'What do I do now?' I thought. The smell of stale urine overpowered me and made my eyes water. I considered putting the sock back on and trying to hide that this had happened; or should I come clean and tell him? I couldn't make a decision so I rolled up the sock with the rest of his belongings, put it in a bag and quickly got out of there to tell his clinician what had just happened. Unfortunately there was no saving that toe. It would have been dead a while to drop off so easily. I was left wondering how someone so smart and successful could have such poor personal hygiene.

Another time, someone came in with chest pain. He was wearing a pristine suit. As I took his trousers off, I saw he had fishnet stockings on with painted red toenails. 'Oh,' I said. 'I like your nail varnish!' I thought it was brilliant. It was the fishnet stockings that got me. There was nothing about him that said 'I dress up like a woman on Thursdays.' I've learnt never to judge by appearances or to take things at face value.

There are the classic stories of people getting things stuck in orifices, of which every A&E professional has hundreds. One man I saw had a carving fork stuck up his anus. He was in his eighties and said he had been experimenting with his wife. I loved his honesty. 'Good on you,' I thought.

Usually you get teenage boys that say: 'I fell on [insert object here].' No one falls at the exact angle and with enough force to get a deodorant can, for example, stuck up their ass. I say deodorant cans, because they are often used – so much so that we once had a discussion trying to guess from the X-ray what brand it was. Vibrators are also popular; once I asked someone how they knew it was still there. He said he could feel it vibrating. This was eight hours later. I was impressed by the long battery life. Sometimes people put animals up there which is a form of cruelty – they usually die.

I love working in A&E. It's a constant sprint, but a marathon at the same time. You're always busy, no one sits down and rests. You're kept on your toes.

The sense of teamwork is amazing. We work as one and there isn't the hierarchy you can sometimes get in other areas. There's no divide between doctors and nurses. It's respectful and everyone trusts one another. When I've got through a shift, I think: 'I've achieved that with a great team.' I go to work for the team. I don't want to let them down and that keeps me going too.

The stuff we see is insane and it's impossible to get bored.

I look back at my career trajectory. Eight years ago, I was a newly qualified nurse, new to the hospital and the city. The opportunities to progress are incredible. You can follow whatever takes your fancy, whether it's clinical advancement, teaching, management or research. I don't think other professions are quite the same.

If you've worked in A&E, you can work almost anywhere. And that's been made even more apparent since this pandemic began. You see the whole range of humanity in the emergency department and I've noticed even more acutely the best and worst parts of human nature in all its raw glory.

2

It's Just in Wuhan

I first heard about coronavirus on the news and from my husband's brother. He was living in China with his wife and used to update us daily on a group chat. He was really blasé about it. 'It's just scaremongering,' he would say. 'They're overreacting.' Every day there'd be more restrictions on his life as they gradually shut down the country until it was total lockdown. 'This is over-kill,' he insisted. 'Not many people have died.'

We kept hearing about his life as the changes took hold. Only one member of the household was allowed out once a day. There were security guards who checked their temperatures when they left the apartment complex. They had a pass to get in and out of their home. They told us they had fostered loads of animals because people were dumping them in the street to get killed.

I started seeing the images of overcrowded hospitals in Wuhan on TV and thought, 'Oh wow, that looks hectic.' It was terrible for them, but I was glad it wasn't in the UK. It was so far away and I never thought that we would be affected. I thought it would spread beyond Wuhan a bit but not to the extent that it ended up blanketing what seemed like the whole world. Perhaps that was me being naive, or perhaps it was a lack of understanding about this new disease.

Although news of the virus was drip-fed into my work and personal worlds, life carried on largely as normal in December and January. I had Christmas off – a rare treat – so spent it with my family. I was working days over the end of December and didn't dare stay up to see the new year in because I liked to be as rested as possible for each shift. Before becoming an ACP I'd found the work had become second nature. It was easy and that's why I wanted to become an ACP. I craved a challenge and to be a better nurse with more time for patients.

When I began in the role, in October 2019, I was as nervous as when I first started in the NHS. Every day was so mentally exhausting. I was constantly on high alert and double checking everything I did while making sure I documented it correctly. I got so worried that if I didn't get enough sleep, it would impact on my work the next day and my ability to care for patients. So I made sure I got at least six, ideally eight, hours' sleep.

Alongside work, everyday life continued. The weather at the beginning of the year was miserable; there were floods, the days were short, the dogs always rolled around in the vast quantities of mud on their walks, and I was feeling more exhausted than usual. Life in A&E is unrelenting.

My dogs mean the world to me. We got Lexie because I wanted company during my days off when Ed was at work. She was a rescue dog, a Labrador cross, and had obviously been abused by a past owner because, when we first got her, she was very nervous and barked at every stranger that came into the house. She still makes a racket when the postman delivers anything. We adopted Max, a Parson terrier, a couple of years later when his owner couldn't look after him anymore. He is a rascal. Leave any food anywhere within his reach and he'll inhale it in seconds. He once destroyed a packet of pistachios my sister had brought and spent the next day pooping whole ones out. He hadn't even chewed them. He also mauled a friend's phone because it smelt of coconut butter handcream.

When I get time off, Ed and I like to go running, especially with the dogs. One Saturday morning, I was driving to a cross country race my running club had asked me to take part in. I hate cross country running but find it hard to say no, so there I was, on my way to what would turn out to be hours of trudging through mud that was so deep and sticky that my left shoe came off.

In the car, a message came through from my sister. It read: 'Are you there?' She was in Brazil for work. She is a journalist and was on a month-long reporting assignment. My sister rarely gets in touch, especially when she is thousands of miles away, and so I knew it was something important. I called her back with the hands-free set in the car. She picked up immediately.

'Hi, Louise. I need some advice,' she said sheepishly.

'Oh, OK. What's up? How was your new year?'

'I'll tell you about that later. Am I on speakerphone?'

'Yes.'

'Is Ed there?'

'Yes, we're on our way to a race.'

'Can you take me off speakerphone please?'

'I can't, I'm driving.'

'Ugh, this is awkward,' she said, addressing the both of us. 'Well, you're my brother-in-law now, so I guess I can tell you.'

Already, worst-case scenarios had started forming in my mind. To give you a brief insight into my sister, she is, what I would describe as, a shit magnet. Bad things happen to her. I say bad, but what I mean is that some of the situations she gets herself into are ridiculous and provide endless entertainment at family get-togethers.

There was the time, when she was learning to drive, that our father asked if she wanted to go to a nearby town for practice. He was very dedicated to her passing her driving test. I think he saw it as a challenge that would keep him entertained and occupied for months. I decided to go along because I had little else to do with my time while living in rural North Yorkshire. Dad went in the passenger seat and I was in the back. We were on the way home when the unexpected happened. I still to this day do not know how, but she somehow managed to stall halfway up a hill that had been immediately preceded by a steep downhill. Panic ensued. Her hands were flailing everywhere, she was screaming and Dad was shouting: 'Never take your hands off the wheel!' Meanwhile, the car was slowly creeping backwards, inching ever closer to the Ferrari that was on our tail. I looked out the back window and made an apologetic face to the driver before turning around and giggling to myself.

When she finally did pass, Dad didn't like her driving all that often. Perhaps he had a premonition of what was to come when she wrote off my mum's car about six months later and only narrowly missed crashing into a very sturdy and unmovable tree.

She got on the wrong train once in France and ended up in Italy. She's missed countless other trains and flights. When it comes to relationships, I would describe her love life as unfortunate. So naturally, when I heard her sheepish voice on the other end of the phone, I started thinking the worst.

'I've got diarrhoea, Louise. It's really bad. I've hardly slept all night. When is it going to stop? I've taken three Immodium tablets and it's eased off slightly,' she said, much to my disappointment.

'You shouldn't take Immodium, you need to let it all pass through your body.'

'I mean, a lot has already come out. Like, a lot. I've been to the toilet I don't know how many times.

It's just as well I've got my own en-suite room now, because I was in a dorm in a hostel the night before last. I'm booked in to go on an eight-hour boat trip today. Is that OK do you think, or am I going to poo my pants?'

'Ooooooh, that could be risky.'

'I've only got a full day on this island and then I'm working. I can't imagine there's much more to come out of my body.'

'OK, well make sure the boat has a toilet and stick to dry crackers for food.'

'OK, thanks. I'll see how I go.'

I guess I felt honoured that she valued my medical advice, given that my parents usually ignored any insights I offered, only to be told exactly the same by the GP. Ed, who had previously lost control of his bowels on a trip with me around India, and I were expecting worse and found the call anticlimactic.

I messaged her later to check on her and she told me she hadn't been able to move far and had got up in the middle of the night to go to the toilet, fainted and hit her head on the tiled floor. I told her to drink more water. The rest of her trip passed without incident, thankfully, and she landed back in the UK safe and sound at the end of the month.

I wasn't to know then that a couple of days later, both our lives would change irrevocably.

* * *

It was Monday 27 January. I had the week off work and had just finished eating supper when my mum called. I picked up and she told me that Dad had passed away. What? Why? How? I started sobbing uncontrollably. I couldn't understand. He was eighty-six but there was nothing wrong with him. We'd been playing silly games and telling Christmas cracker jokes only a month before. I sat on the sofa stunned and shocked, and wept. Lexie knew something was wrong and she didn't leave my side.

The next morning, I went up to North Yorkshire with Ed to be with my mum. My sister was due in from London later on that morning. I went to meet her at the train station. She got off the train, and started crying as she walked towards me before she hugged me. She never hugs me, and I can't remember the last time I saw her cry.

The next few days were a mix of dark humour, tears and country walks. Ed, a news junkie, kept us informed of all the latest coronavirus developments in China but that was the last thing on all our minds.

Mum told us how Dad died. The pair of them had just finished supper and were about to watch the evening news. He was sitting in his favourite chair when he suddenly started fitting. Blood came out of his mouth. Mum told us of her struggle to get him on the floor to perform CPR. She called for an ambulance. The paramedics arrived and worked on him for forty-five minutes. It sounded like he had gone very quickly and no amount of resuscitation was going to bring him back.

In a way we were all grateful that his life ended like that. It was quick and he was spared a long, slow and painful death. It didn't make the gut-wrenching grief any easier, though. I wondered when I had last spoken to him. I frantically searched through my calls history and emails to see what I'd last said to him. All I wanted to do was to talk to him again.

I had often thought that Dad dying would see us all around his bed arguing over when to stop life support. I always believed his decline would be gradual and that I would see it coming and be able to have some medical input. But this was so out of my control and the last thing that I thought would have happened. We decided against a post-mortem so I don't know exactly what Dad died of but I've gone over and over his last moments in my head, trying to understand medically what happened. Accepting I will never have an answer has been incredibly hard but I do know there was no way anyone would have been able to save him.

Throughout those days, I never saw Mum cry. She kept herself busy. We all got on with sorting out the mountain of admin that comes when someone dies. Death has never been a taboo subject in my family, and Dad had prepared a folder with instructions on what to do on 'his passing'. He'd even written his own tribute; it was terrible, very dry, and read a bit like a cover letter for a job with a truncated list of some of his achievements. My sister offered to have a go at re-writing it with Mum's help. I was so impressed by the end result and how she delivered it with such confidence in the church. The whole congregation was captivated. It was beautifully written and a fantastic portrayal of Dad's life. That period ended up bringing us closer together as sisters.

After the initial shock had passed, I felt, along with my sister, that we should thank the paramedics for being so diligent and for staying with my mum for far longer than they needed to. Dad would have been so appreciative too. I know how hard some cases can be, particularly when you then have to move on to the next patient and continue your shift. When we get thanks, it's often because of a life saved but unfortunately in this case, it was my father's time. I tracked down an email address and sent a message to the ambulance crew. It was reassuring to have my wider colleagues show first-hand how amazing our NHS emergency team is, and how valuable we are to families and society.

That time immediately after his passing was a bit of a blur. My emotions washed over me like waves; one minute I'd be fine and then the next floored with grief. It was exhausting. There were moments of light relief, though. My mum, sister and I were sitting together in the lounge one evening when my mum asked my sister about 'her man'.

'What's this?' I asked.

'It's nothing,' she replied, before launching into a detailed description of the crush she had formed on someone she had never spoken to. I don't know how she gets herself into these situations.

'Honestly, it's pathetic. How old are you?' Mum said, teasing her. 'Was it a Master's you got and now you can't even say hello to someone? You're acting like a spotty teenager!'

There was one night we all got drunk and opened the door to a neighbour who had come to drop off a condolences card. And I remember trying to wash my dead father's blood out of the cushions from his favourite chair. I stood at the kitchen sink and thought aloud: 'I never thought I'd be doing this.' That chair has remained empty ever since.

At the weekend, my sister went back to London. Ed had returned to work some days before so it was just me and Mum for a little while. We both teared up when I left. Dad had said he wanted to be cremated and Mum had agreed with him that we would hold a service of thanksgiving to celebrate his life and mourn his passing. Both the cremation and the service were to happen on 12 February.

During the days in between, I was taken aback by the strength of my grief. One day, it took me five hours to get up off the upstairs landing floor. I don't even remember how I got there in the first place. I'm normally very proactive and can't sit through an entire film without feeling the need to be doing something else, so to be caught in this state of paralysis came as a shock to me.

When I finally made it out of the house to the launderette (our utility room was being refurbished and so the washing machine was unplugged), I sat watching the repetitive circular motion of my laundry for forty-five minutes while crying. It was the type of sobbing where you struggle to breathe. I had palpitations and felt so uncomfortable being outside. I couldn't pick up the phone to friends who were calling me as the thought of talking to them was unbearable.

It wasn't long before I had to decide what to do about work. How long is an appropriate time to take off when your father dies? My sister returned to work after a week. I was jealous and angry that she had managed to regain some form of normality, but then I remembered what was expected of me.

Officially, we get two days' leave for a bereavement of a close family member. If you need longer, you get signed off work, ill. The thought of people dying in front of me when my grief was so raw made me feel sick with worry, so I decided to take some time out. I was also worried that my patient care would be compromised and didn't want any lives put at unnecessary risk.

I wasn't ready to make decisions about whether resuscitating a patient whose heart had stopped was in their best interests, or for the difficult and frank conversations I would inevitably have to have with patients and families. I didn't want to have to break bad news, like the time I had to tell a patient that the back pain they'd had for the last six months – and I had to stop myself from rolling my eyes when they were first admitted – was a symptom of their as yet undiagnosed lung cancer which had spread to the spine. I couldn't muster the energy to be my usual, upbeat self.

After the initial all-encompassing fog of grief lifted, I realized I had an advanced life support refresher course coming up at work. It involved a written and practical exam. You're a very fortunate person if you manage to get on to these courses and they're in high demand and very expensive.

Not wanting to disappoint, I decided to return to work. The written test was fine. In the practical exam we were given a simulation scenario which had already been scripted. The one assigned to me led to me having to make the difficult but correct decision to stop resuscitating the patient. Everyone else managed to save a life. Typical, I thought. Straight afterwards, I burst into tears. It was too close to home and the whole team knew it. They were really nice about it, though, and gathered round me to give me some comfort and to let me know I'd handled it really well.

My first shift back on the shop floor of A&E involved comforting the daughter of a patient who we had decided to complete a Do Not Attempt Resuscitation (DNAR) form on. She completely agreed with the decision but seeing her sobbing and whimpering 'Dad' as she sat by his bedside was heart-wrenching and emotionally testing for me. My next patient had taken an overdose because their father had died that day. The saying 'bad luck comes in threes' certainly seemed true at that moment.

As the weeks passed, I still thought about Dad every day, more than I thought about Covid-19. The threat from the virus didn't seem real, unlike the pain of losing Dad. Even when I found out about one of the first cases of suspected Covid-19 in Newcastle, I still didn't really take it seriously. We were told in a meeting at work, but the sentiment was very much one of, 'We'll be fine, guys.' I thought that Newcastle was fairly distant. My mother was in North Yorkshire but a good hour and a half drive away, and my sister was in London. Then, on 12 February, the first case in the capital was confirmed, a woman who'd returned from China. By 27 February the UK had 15 confirmed cases.

In hindsight, my dad had impeccable timing in dying when he did. It was the same when he was alive. He had been a colonel in the army and our childhood was dominated by his teachings on timekeeping, integrity, charm, tidiness, and 'work hard, play hard' approach to life. Not all of it rubbed off on my sister; despite her being intelligent and highly capable, tidiness is not her strong point. I used to get paid £5 to find her glasses in her mess of a bedroom.

Dad would have been classed in the vulnerable, high-risk group of people most susceptible to the damaging effects of this new virus. A natural extrovert, he would have hated physical distancing and not being able to go out and make jokes with all the villagers and the shopkeepers in the nearest town. And if he'd caught the virus? Clinicians across the world were making morally difficult decisions about their patients' care. Deciding who would be taken to intensive care in the hope that they recover and who would not when this escalation in care would prove futile. For some patients, it was simply too late and the best we could do was to make them comfortable.

I know that any medic looking at my dad would have seen a man in his eighties, albeit fit for his age, and would most likely have decided not to escalate him to intensive care. Knowing that is difficult. So, well done, Dad, on dying when you did. As ever, your timing was perfect.

3

It's Here

The beginning of March was still business as usual in A&E. People were coming into the department with little to no concerns regarding coronavirus. The total number of confirmed cases in England on 2 March reached 104. The numbers were small.

Covid-19 was getting closer but I still wasn't overly alarmed yet. I had something else to worry about. I phoned home for a catch-up with Mum one evening; I was really concerned about her living on her own in the house she had shared with my father for so many years. It seemed empty to my sister and me without his presence when we were at home for the cremation and service of thanksgiving. He was such a stable rock in all our lives. She mentioned that her brother, my only uncle, had been diagnosed with lung cancer. She didn't go into detail and said that she hadn't read his email properly, but she did say that an operation was scheduled for a few weeks' time. He'd known when he came up to see us when my father died and had said nothing; I guess it wasn't the right time. That he was having an operation meant that the cancer was localized to one area that they could remove, so I was hopeful. He had also looked well when I saw him. It was another blow to my family though, and so soon into 2020. I hoped my aunt wasn't too worried.

In those early days, I saw a patient who had recently had a nose job. She had gone to Thailand to get it done, which was on the list of countries that were listed as coronavirus hotspots.

'I couldn't afford to have it done in the UK so I had to go abroad,' she said.

Now, she was experiencing swelling and pain.

'Are you experiencing any other symptoms?' I asked her. I was a little wary that she might have coronavirus.

'I haven't had a fever, a cough or a sore throat, if that's what you're getting at. I definitely don't have the coronavirus.'

Those symptoms were the warning signs at the time. I asked my specialist ear, nose and throat colleague to come and review her as I knew next to nothing about nose jobs. He shared my anxiety, but I reassured him that she had no Covid symptoms. Little did I know then that so many people would be carriers of the virus while presenting no symptoms.

Face masks were hardly used at the time so it was a surprise to walk into one cubicle and see a woman wearing one with unicorns and rainbows all over it. It seemed like a fashion statement, especially when she took it off when I stepped in to see her. Was I a safe bet? I tried to suppress the 6 a.m. sniffles that I get most night shifts when I've been working for hours and am tired.

The first real case of definite Covid-19 I saw was a patient in her forties, at the end of the first week in March. The first person in England died on 5 March after testing positive for coronavirus. Italy, meanwhile, was in crisis. By 6 March, their death toll had grown sixfold in six days; more than 230 Italians were dead and caseloads were growing by more than 1,200 every day. My patient had attended A&E because she was feeling short of breath. None of us was wearing personal protective equipment (PPE) at that time, apart from a cursory apron and pair of gloves. I remember looking at her chest X-ray and a colleague glancing over my shoulder and saying, 'Well that's a terrible-looking chest.' It was odd because she had evidence of a potential infection in both of her lungs. I assumed it was pneumonia, but that usually only presents in one lung, not two. Little did I know at the time that her chest X-ray was what I would come to recognize as an obvious sign that the virus had embedded itself in someone.

She was none the wiser to Covid. She'd recently travelled, but not to one of the areas that were on the news. When I look back, all the clues were there and it was obvious. She was barely conscious, her eyes weren't open and her breathing was very laboured. When patients aren't able to talk, I just get on with my job. I don't start a conversation expecting them to talk back to me because they're so exhausted and I need them to conserve energy. It was obvious she needed to go to intensive care so I called them and they came straight down. It was the ICU doctor who told me bilateral signs of consolidation on a chest X-ray was a sign of Covid. My heart sank into the pit of my stomach. 'It's here,' I thought.

We weren't immune anymore and it had come to us. My thoughts went deep down a rabbit hole; this was the start of a long battle. I'd heard what my brother-in-law had been experiencing in China and thought that would be us. We wouldn't be able to go anywhere. China had built a new hospital in six or seven days. We couldn't do that, so what the hell were we going to do? I thought about the images I had seen of mass graves. Our mortuary had reached capacity one winter and a makeshift extension was erected to house all the bodies. If that happened in one winter, how were we going to deal with a pandemic?

This was getting dark and I began to feel that I was pre-empting things and being a bit too negative. 'Chill out, Louise,' I told myself. We hadn't even got her swab result back yet so it wasn't like we knew for sure. I didn't have any thoughts at the time about me being infected. She hadn't coughed on me and we're so used to dealing with infections that it didn't really cross my mind. Perhaps it was because it was before we knew just how easily it spread. We found out she did test positive; the news went round the department like wildfire. It wasn't long before coronavirus was our new normal, however, and stopped being newsworthy in our professional lives.

The following night, a disgruntled man in his twenties came in accompanied by an entourage of police officers – six in total. Wasn't this a bit excessive?

'What's brought you to A&E this evening?' I asked before he threw his shoes across the room, and then looked around to see what else he could launch in my direction. I couldn't help glancing towards a sharps bin in the corner where the scissors and scalpels had been disposed of, and was so glad of those six officers when they reacted quickly and restrained him.

Violence is part and parcel of working in A&E, unfortunately. I've had a long list of insults yelled at me that I won't bore you with here. Once I heard a drunk patient shouting and ran to find him ripping off his monitoring, throwing thousands of pounds' worth of equipment across the room.

'What are you doing?' I asked in what I thought was a perfectly reasonable manner. He came and stood one centimetre away from my face and said, 'I'm going to kill you.' He reached into his pocket, but before I knew it, one of my colleagues had restrained him up against the wall.

I'm lucky; in some cases, the violence can be extreme. There have been healthcare professionals who have been injured or even killed. We're often threatened with rape and spat at. One of my colleagues was screamed at and hit around the head when she asked someone to move out of the way so she could pass with an elderly patient in a wheelchair.

One afternoon a few years ago, I had a visit from two police officers saying they had received a call from a man who was threatening to kill me. He had mentioned me by name after he'd glanced at my badge when I was treating him in the department. He had been discharged and later decided to ring the police. I laughed it off, telling myself that if he really wanted to kill me, he wouldn't have informed the police of his intention to do so. Even so, it didn't stop me glancing over my shoulder as I left work that evening.

I assessed my latest violent patient and deemed him safe for discharge back to police custody. As he was being escorted out of the hospital, he started shouting, 'I'VE GOT THE CORONAVIRUS.' We all laughed nervously and tried to give reassuring smiles to the patients he passed.

Later that week, Covid started to loom larger over A&E and everyone's minds. It seemed to go from nothing to everything in quite a short amount of time. By 10 March, a sixth person had died in the UK and the number of confirmed cases was at 373. There were bound to be many others though, because there wasn't widespread testing at that point. Airlines cancelled all flights to and from Italy as the Italian government's decision to put the entire country on lockdown came into effect. I'd just booked a holiday in Pembrokeshire at the end of April to celebrate my birthday. It's strange when I look back at how I was planning normal life right up until lockdown changed everything.

A few days later, the department was turned completely upside down. A&E spread across almost an entire floor of the hospital, taking over many other clinics, in order to create capacity. We had an isolation unit with around ten beds, and there was a Covid resuscitation area on top of that with nine beds. The department was split into hot and cold areas. Hot was coronavirus, cold was everything else. We were running two A&Es because we still needed a resuscitation area, and a minors and majors part of the department for those patients who weren't infected and needed to be kept that way. (Minors is our shorthand for the walking wounded – people with a minor illness or injury – and majors means those with more acute problems who come in on a trolley.)

A few days later I had a meeting with all my ACP colleagues where we were told that our shift patterns were changing. With three days' notice, my entire rota had been completely rewritten. Most of it now comprised of shifts that finished at midnight, or night shifts where I would finish at 8 a.m. Afterwards, we tried to cheer ourselves up with the thought of all the extra pennies we would be earning by working unsociable hours; ones that would be saved for when this was all over. At least I didn't have child care to juggle amid all this chaos. It did present a bit of a challenge for the dogs, though. Our dog walker had stopped working because of the coronavirus situation and as I was starting later in the day, I was the one that had to take them out. They need a lot of exercise. I used to have dog-walking as a back-up career dream plan. That soon became a little less attractive when waking up early every day for weeks on end to take them out lost its novelty.

I've got a bad sense of direction too, something that runs in the family, and often got lost on my own with the dogs. One day I found myself having to phone my husband at work because I kept finding myself back at the same junction in some cruel *Groundhog Day* nightmare. I'd already been out for three hours and even the dogs were tired. I also had no snacks on me, for me or the dogs. His work colleagues were in fits of laughter as they heard him trying to calm an emotional and hungry wife. I sometimes resented having to walk the dogs so much but, in truth, being surrounded by nature's beauty and peace really did make a positive change. And I needed those moments where my brain could rest as our whole way of working was turned on its head. Policies started to change, we made major alterations to where we would send patients in the hospital. We were having more discussions with every department in the hospital. We were learning a whole new disease process as well as how to detect it, diagnose and manage it. This was work I'd never had to do before – learning to interpret the chest X-ray of a Covid patient, how to turn a patient in respiratory difficulty onto their front to improve their breathing. It was all completely alien to me. I was still learning months into the pandemic because no one really knew how to manage it. It was all so new and there wasn't enough evidence. As each day went by, the death toll would rise and new evidence would come out guiding towards a different way of managing the virus.

That aspect of guesswork was perhaps part of what made this whole situation all the more terrifying for me.

Let me explain. I've had patients who come into A&E when they really don't need to. One girl once came in with a spot.

'Genuinely, what do you want me to do?' I asked.

'What is it?' she said.

'It's a spot,' I told her. 'It's not a problem that we in A&E are best equipped to help with.' People also came in with a common cold. GPs get annoyed when that happens, let alone us.

A&E is so readily available. It's great because you come in and essentially we give you a bit of an MOT and tell you what's wrong or not wrong. That's some-times all people want but it can stop us from giving timely care to those that need it most. We don't help ourselves because we continue to do it. As well as anxieties about our patients, we have the threat of litigation hanging over us like a guillotine ready to take off our head.

I struggled with this in my first months as an ACP more than ever before. I was newly qualified. I didn't have the experience or the confidence to not check absolutely everything that I could to make sure that I was doing the right thing.

'One day you will kill a patient,' I was always told in my training. I think what they meant was that I'd potentially miss a diagnosis and the patient would die. I always have that in the back of my mind and it has stopped me from becoming cocky and over confident, but it has also put the fear of God into me.

By this time in March, five months into the job, two patients had already contacted the trust to complain about decisions I had made. It usually happens months down the line. A consultant came up to me when I was working on the shop floor. I was completely oblivious and they asked, 'Do you remember this patient?' It's like asking, 'Can you remember this time when you were three years old?' Then I read the notes and I remembered. They went through everything with me. Luckily, in both situations, I was right in what I had done. But I never know when the day will come when I've done something wrong. As a result, I've learnt to talk to people to try and understand what their expectations and concerns are, because that way I can usually get to the root of the problem. Many want to know they haven't got cancer, or had a heart attack, but it can take a while to get them to articulate their concerns. When they do, usually I can help.

With coronavirus, however, it was all different. From what I was seeing in patients, I knew it could overpower someone so rapidly. They went from being fine to suddenly not in the space of fifteen minutes. My anxiety was off the scale when I saw someone who had symptoms but looked all right. We couldn't keep everyone in hospital so I assessed everything and if they seemed OK, I sent them home with advice to come back if their symptoms worsened. Covid-19 is a respiratory illness so everyone was breathless. How does someone who is not a healthcare professional know when their oxygen levels are dangerously low? They don't. It's different if you've got low blood pressure, say, because you feel dizzy and light-headed. Or, you collapse.

I would feel absolutely dreadful if I found out that my actions had harmed a patient. It hadn't happened yet, but I knew it might be around the corner. It was a sense of foreboding that was always with me. And as coronavirus took hold, that feeling of doom loomed even larger. Nobody knew enough about Covid. I certainly didn't. I spent my time off reading research papers and articles. I couldn't escape from it. I felt fatigued and saturated with information that kept changing. It was guesswork, educated guesswork. I hoped I was doing the right thing by my patients and would often check with my consultant if I had the slightest doubt.

The weekend of 15 March, I had a twenty-mile race. Half marathons had become quite easy for me and I had booked this because I wanted to push myself. Ed was also taking part. I had secretly hoped it might be cancelled because I had never run this far before and I hadn't trained nearly as much as I should have. We drove there and picked up another member of our running club on the way. It was a sunny day and Ed, who is very sensitive to the sun, started sneezing. We all started joking about how he might have coronavirus, but was our guest a bit worried? I couldn't tell for sure.

All other races had been cancelled because of worries around coronavirus. Standing at the beginning and waiting to go felt very different. Normally, it's very crowded and everyone jostles for space, rubbing shoulders. On this occasion, every time someone coughed, there was a moment of tension and audible gasps. I tried desperately to suppress the tickle in my throat.

Ed is a faster runner than me and this race was in the middle of the countryside with no people. It would be lonely and I knew it would just be me in a mental battle with my thoughts for the whole way. My usual running playlist had become too predictable and I wasn't sure it would get me through to the finish line, so I opted for one on Spotify called 'Coronavirus playlist'. Best decision ever. As I ran, I was buoyed by hits such as Nelly's 'Hot in Here' and 'Fever' by Peggy Lee. That soundtrack kept me going until mile sixteen, which is where I hit a block – 'the wall' as many runners term it. Thoughts of not being able to finish crept into my head. I had rationed out jelly sweets to keep track of how many miles I had done. I had two left; one for each two miles. I stopped to walk for a bit because the pain in my legs and joints was getting unbearable, but then I thought that would take me twice as long so I may as well run it. My energy levels were low. It was hard. It was emotional. But I did it and the wave of relief when I finished was palpable, so were the tears. Ed was there waiting. 'Marathon next?' he asked.

The following week cinemas closed, which was truly gutting as I went almost every week with Ed to see the new releases. The day after, Parkrun – a 5km run at 9 a.m. every Saturday that happened in locations around the UK and the rest of the world – was cancelled, which was another blow as it was a weekly feature in our social lives. It was free, open to anyone and everyone, and was a feel-good event and a great start to the day. Well, for my husband and me it was. We even did the local Parkrun the morning of our marriage ceremony. I remember dragging my sister along a couple of times and she hated them, though she did come to cheer with my parents when we ran the 5km on our wedding day.

It was meant to be a colleague's wedding in late March. Her dad had died suddenly of cancer a couple of years ago and her mum had also been diagnosed with cancer. She got engaged in summer 2019 and the wedding was planned for March so that her mother would definitely be there to see her only daughter get married.

The bride-to-be was worried about whether it should go ahead. Her mother was immunocompromised and the majority of the guest list was people who worked in A&E surrounded by lots of germs. It was this awful turmoil; should she potentially expose her mum? She needed to get married because she wanted her mum to see it.

In the end the decision was made for her. Lockdown was announced on 23 March. People were allowed out for essentials like food and medicine, and for exercise close to their home once a day, but that was it. Weddings were definitely not allowed. She decided to have a celebration on the day over Zoom. Everybody posted pictures of themselves in wedding attire, raising a glass to the couple. It was really fun, even if some people only dressed up their top halves that could be seen on screen. Earlier in the day, I had driven round to her house and left a hamper I had put together full of goodies on her doorstep. She later made a new wedding invitation which features a picture of all of us on Zoom for a date in 2021.

As the days and weeks went on, fortieth and ninetieth birthday parties were cancelled, another wedding was postponed. I resisted meeting up with my mum for Mother's Day, though I was quite upset about it. My sister had made it up to Yorkshire before lockdown was announced to work from home and to be with Mum whose grief was still so raw. Self-isolating would be tough enough for anyone, let alone a grieving seventy-year-old widow. I was incredibly grateful to my sister for moving home and being such a rock for my mum during this unsettling time. We had planned a social-distancing picnic, but Mum didn't think it a good idea. She was right. How long would it be before I saw her again?

When I arrived on shift, everyone would come together in a room just off-site with the consultant in charge who discussed where everyone would be working: hot (coronavirus) isolation units or resus, or cold (non coronavirus) minors, majors or resus. I liked this. Before, everyone came in at different times so I'd often be the only one starting at a certain hour. I'd sneak in and tell the consultant I had arrived. This way was better for team morale and there was a stronger feeling of camaraderie.

The consultant would make sure you were suitable to work in the hot area, that you didn't have any risk factors that made you more vulnerable and that you had been fit tested for the masks so that you were safe to work in the area.

Each member of staff underwent a fit test. When I did it, I wore a mask with a hood over my head. A foul-tasting aerosol was sprayed into the hood while I was asked to do various manoeuvres like moving my head up and down, and to the side. I had to talk, and do various breathing techniques. If you can taste the spray, you've failed because it shows the mask wasn't working properly. I passed.

Then there was donning (putting on) and doffing (taking off) the PPE every shift. The first time I wore it, my nose was very sore and bruised. Before you enter an isolation unit, there is a step-by-step process you have to go through. First you wash your hands, then you put on a pair of gloves, a full-sleeved apron which is tied at the back, a respirator and either goggles or a full visor. Lastly you put on a second pair of gloves. Once you've got the process down, it takes a few minutes.

I felt safer when I had PPE on. In cold majors the patients were supposedly not meant to have Covid. A handful of times, when I went to see them, I took an in-depth medical history during which they explained that they had symptoms which were in line with having coronavirus. By that time, I had been in there and examined them, potentially exposing myself for around twenty minutes.

In that way, PPE made me feel more secure; all I had to do was remove my top pair of gloves and extra apron after each patient. That didn't mean it wasn't so uncomfortable though. Even having a conversation would lead to me getting out of breath, and I like to think I'm quite fit. When giving patients advice, I'd have to stop mid-sentence to catch my breath. I was always hot and everything felt like so much effort. With the mask across my face and a visor coming down over the front, I felt so claustrophobic.

Going to the toilet was a nightmare. You'd have to

be so careful about doffing the PPE, making sure you took it off so that you didn't touch any areas that had been exposed and that you disposed of it correctly. Then, because a one-way system had been introduced to reduce cross-contamination from hot and cold areas, I had to walk a long way round to get to the bathroom. It became a fifteen-minute trip, instead of the two minutes it normally took. I often ended up waiting till my break for periods of time of up to six or seven hours.

Doffing the PPE at the end of a shift was a laborious process. Each time I came out of an isolation unit, I would peel it off and away from me. I washed my hands before I touched anything on my face. Last to come off was the mask. I couldn't fling it off my face but took the straps off away from my head, held them out in front and then dropped the mask into the bin. Hand washing followed each individual step. Often, by the end of a shift, my hands would be so dry, they'd start to crack.

Inside the isolation unit, I always wrote my name on my apron because much of my face was covered and I couldn't even recognize my own colleagues. The PPE made conveying empathy and compassion to patients more difficult. This is such a vital part of patient care that was missing and made this new virus all the more cruel and inhumane. The mask goes right up to beneath your eyes so no one could tell if you were smiling or pulling another facial expression. It's harder to be heard and I had to make sure I enunciated every letter at a louder volume. It was tiring to constantly repeat things over and over again.

If appropriate I'd put my hand near the patient to show a level of comfort, or I'd put my arm on their trolley. It must have been so scary for patients so I made more of an effort when I went in to see them. I told them I was smiling and made a joke about how they couldn't see it. I hope I went some way to easing their distress and panic.

Before Covid hit, I was used to feeling pretty confident in my surroundings at work. I was often the nurse in charge of certain areas. It's often said that nurses are the backbone of the NHS; I certainly felt that was the case. If anybody needed anything, I would normally have the answer. I knew all the protocols and where everything was. If I didn't know the answer I knew someone that did. In the isolation unit, however, everything was new and I felt like I was stepping into the unknown. I realized how junior doctors who constantly do rotations must feel when they have to start over in a new department or hospital. I didn't know where anything was. I felt stressed because there were new protocols and it was overwhelming. All my previous knowledge was almost useless in this new environment. I think everybody felt like this to some extent.

There was more though. I was only a few months into my new role and wasn't completely at home yet with the increased responsibility I had. Clinical decision-making was new to me and it was scary. Anxieties around whether I was doing the right thing were ever present. Was the man in front of me constipated or had he got an obstruction with a potential bowel perforation?

At the beginning, the symptoms of Covid were fairly defined so we knew who should be in isolation. We'd later find out that there were other symptoms of course. Was someone's temperature more than 37.8, had they had a persistent cough in the last seven days?

Patients were kept in the isolation unit for hours at first, which was too long. I had one patient who was waiting for a bed on a ward for twelve hours. This was because the public hadn't grasped how serious the situation might become and we were still getting the high numbers that normally came to A&E. It very quickly changed, however; I would ask for a bed on a ward and five minutes later, there would be one. That was unheard of. Management had made it happen as they didn't want people hanging around in A&E for fear of the virus spreading.

One man was surprised he had the virus when the test came back positive. 'I haven't left the house in three weeks!' he exclaimed.

'Have you got any family?' I asked.

'No.'

'Who has been helping you with your shopping?' He was in his eighties and couldn't walk more than a few metres.

'My niece has been coming in most days, but she's been feeling fine, so it can't be her.'

I didn't know who else could have transmitted the virus, but I didn't want to point the finger of blame at anyone. We were beyond the point of contact tracing. It was starting to feel like the situation had got out of control.

After six back-to-back shifts working in isolation, I was tired. I went into the roll call we had at the beginning of each shift thinking that if I was going to be put in the Covid area again, I would have to say something. I hate to be someone who makes a fuss and I often just get on with things but I was getting desperate. The consultant came in and asked, 'Right, who has worked two shifts in isolation?' My hand shot up. Some others had too. He went round the room asking how long each person had worked in the Covid areas. When it got to me and I said I'd done six shifts in there, everybody turned round and looked at me aghast. The consultant said, 'Right, you can have a break then.' I was so pleased to have a day working in non-Covid minors. It was a welcome rest for my face, which had suffered while I wore a respirator mask that pinched the bridge of my nose and cheeks. It also made me feel like an overweight hippopotamus when I climbed the stairs and tried to talk at the same time.

A&E had become very quiet very quickly once the virus seeped into everyone's consciousness. We'd normally have between 600 and 700 patients a day but admissions to the department had halved, which was worrying in itself. Were people suffering at home when they didn't need to be? That day on the non-Covid minors section I was reminded there were still patients out there who were on the hypochondriac end of the spectrum.

I saw one woman in her fifties who had skipped lunch, stood up quickly after watching television, felt dizzy and ended up crawling her way to the kitchen where her partner was. She had given her a chocolate bar and some lemonade and she immediately felt better.

'Do you think it's a heart attack, doctor?' she asked.

No, I didn't. Nevertheless, I carried out all the necessary urgent investigations to reassure her that she had not had a heart attack. After half an hour, I told her, 'All your test results have come back fine. You're ready to be discharged now.'

'Are you sure there's nothing wrong with me?'

'I've done a thorough examination and your results suggest everything is as it should be.'

'Is there anything I need to do to make sure I don't end up back in A&E?'

'Definitely don't skip any meals in future,' I said.

My next patient was middle-aged and had been sent in by her GP with a swollen, red, hot and painful calf. The GP had put her on a course of antibiotics; they thought it might be an infection. There had been no improvement after five days and so here she was. I was flummoxed. I had no idea how to manage a patient in this way; this is normally a complaint handled in primary care and not A&E. I spent an hour and a half on the phone to various different people arranging an ultrasound and follow-up appointment for her, as well as writing a prescription for the right drug for a blood clot in her leg. I was desperately trying not to feel annoyed at what was most likely a severely overstretched GP practice. Then I spent a further thirty minutes teaching her how to inject herself with the drug as nobody would be able to come out to her over the next couple of days.

I went to see another patient who had a fungating tumour on her left breast. It was really difficult to mask the look of shock and horror on my face when I peeled back her shirt and saw it. It also smelt really bad and my eyes were watering. She had been diagnosed with cancer shortly after her son had passed away. She had to be admitted to hospital. I referred her to the oncology department who told me her recent scans showed a spread of the cancer that was inoperable. She would be told the next day that nothing more could be done. Awful things were still happening to good people, outside of the pandemic.

My time of relative respite in the cold area didn't last any longer as my consultant came up to me in a hurry. 'Louise, I need you to go and work in isolation again. Can you make your way there now please?' I wasn't even halfway through my shift when I found myself back in PPE and in the unit of claustrophobia.

They would have sent the other doctor on shift, but he had a young baby at home.

By late March there was clear messaging over what to do if you had come into contact with someone who had recently returned from a country where the virus was prolific. Although advice was changing, I thought it was pretty obvious that you were to isolate at home if you had the following symptoms: a dry cough, a temperature or shortness of breath. We'd put huge signs up at every entrance to the hospital explaining when you should be self-isolating.

Yet still, some of the patients I saw were oblivious to what was going on around them. The media were reporting only one story – coronavirus – and the death toll in England was getting higher with each passing day. Did people not read or watch the news? Had they not seen the signs up everywhere or even heard the general chit-chat on the streets?

One day, I walked into the isolation unit to see a patient. He told me he had a cough and a fever but assured me he hadn't travelled recently. I continued taking his medical history. It all tallied with suspected coronavirus.

'Just to double check, you definitely haven't travelled abroad in the last few weeks; or been in contact with anyone who has?' I asked.

'Oh yeah, I've been looking after my friend who was unwell after returning from China.'

The country, China, where this whole thing started, did he mean? It had taken twenty minutes to get to this point. And he had gone into the main A&E before he was transferred to the isolation unit.

I felt frustration building but knew I had to keep a lid on it. I reminded myself that sometimes people aren't exposed to the news; maybe they weren't aware of all the guidelines about what to do if you started getting symptoms? It was my role to educate people and not to be judgemental. Sometimes it's really hard though. Especially when this man had put who knew how many other people at risk just by coming into A&E that day.

I explained the gravity of the situation and that we needed to try to prevent the spread of the virus. He was well enough to go home and self-isolate. I told him what to look out for that would indicate when he should come back in to hospital.

'Do you live with anybody?' I asked.

'No,' he replied.

'How are you going to get home?' was my next question.

'Oh, I'll get my sister to come and pick me up.'

I'm not totally sure he had understood what I had said about how viruses spread. I felt exasperated.

You'll sometimes get patients coming in with a diarrhoea and vomiting bug only to see their family trundle in to visit them, touching everything before consuming a takeaway meal they'd snuck in for the patient. The next day they'd be back with the same bug and wondering how they had got it. This is how diseases spread. Hand hygiene is such a basic and effective tool, yet too often neglected.

Some minutes later, a student nurse who was shadowing me said he had a sore throat. 'You'd best go home,' I told him. Government advice at the time stated that if you had flu-like symptoms you had to stay at home for seven days. This applied to healthcare professionals as well, because, just like the rest of the population, we didn't have access to testing. It led to a huge amount of staff having to be off work, and within A&E there weren't the usual amount of nursing staff on duty. The ones that came in were stretched. In these situations, where there is increased pressure on everyone, people can get ratty and short tempered. I'd help out every way I was able to try and keep team morale up.

4

A Mental Health Crisis

I was in A&E writing up my patient's notes when I heard the familiar sounds of someone in mental distress. The police often bring people in crisis to the emergency department because it is considered a safe place to keep someone until they are in a calmer state. We also have a great mental health team. I couldn't make out what this woman was shouting, but I detected the odd 'virus' in amidst a torrent of words. I went to see her but couldn't make any sense of what she was saying, let alone perform much of an examination. She was so distressed that security arrived to help keep us and her safe.

When people are in a mental health crisis, they can sometimes lash out at anyone in the way. Sometimes that's us healthcare workers; we can be perceived as a threat. We shouldn't really be victims of any violence in our workplace but I can understand and forgive these people because I know that what they have been through to get into this state must have been truly traumatic.

I could see she was transfixed by her phone. She kept staring at it.

'What's that you keep looking at? Can I take a look?'

On the screen was a list of words. 'Wash hands' was written over and over again. I found her husband's number in her phone and rang him. He was shocked, telling me she was fine yesterday – 'her normal self', he said. 'She seemed to be behaving a little oddly this morning,' he added, 'but I didn't think anything of it and dropped her off at work.'

'What does she do?'

'She's a supermarket delivery driver.'

A change in behaviour can be a result of an infection, electrolyte imbalance, drugs, toxins, a bleed on the brain, or mental health problems. She had no history of mental illness so I took bloods, an ECG and a CT scan of her head. All returned normal. I was perplexed. What could have caused this sudden change in behaviour?

By then, she'd been with us for around three hours and was beginning to show signs of settling down. I called the mental health team who assessed her. Afterwards, they told me they had diagnosed her with stress-induced psychosis. She had been so concerned about contracting and transmitting the virus through her day job that it had led to her going into crisis mode. I knew about the effect stress could have on people, but this was a whole new level.

It was incredibly worrying that somebody could

become so acutely unwell from stress brought on by the pandemic. Not only that, but this woman had been exposed to radiation when we scanned her brain, a step we only take if absolutely necessary. So much time and resources had been taken up to investigate what could be wrong and then, after everything, she recovered within five hours. I had never seen anything like this.

This episode showed me that coronavirus would have a much bigger impact than I originally thought. It wasn't just those who were infected that might suffer with their health. I feared we would see a lot more anxiety-related problems in A&E and I was right. Over the next few weeks and months, there was a spike in mental health attendances; more people were coming in with chest pain that was anxiety-related.

While a lot of our 'regulars' – those who we'd often see multiple times a week in the department presenting with the same complaint – dropped off, new people were coming in.

I could understand why. Even in my circle of my friends, people were struggling. Some were losing their jobs, or being furloughed. Our dog-walker wasn't working at the moment and I wondered how she was managing. People were trapped at home unable to do many things that they enjoyed and that helped them manage some of the dark times in their life. There was so much economic instability; the stock markets were all over the place. If my dad had been alive, this would have been a major cause for concern for him. He loved talking about the stock market.

It wasn't just the general population's mental health that was worsening, either.

I read a news story that said an intensive care nurse who was treating Covid-19 patients had killed herself. I knew that coronavirus wouldn't be the only reason and that she probably had underlying mental health problems, but it seemed as though everything bad was being linked to the virus. There was overwhelming sadness everywhere.

It was amazing how quickly the messaging around coronavirus changed, even within the hospital. Right at the beginning when there were only a few cases, the trust would send an email that went a little bit like this:

'You may have heard in the media that we've had two deaths linked to coronavirus. Both were in their 80s and 90s with underlying health conditions.'

'Underlying health conditions' became a part of the lexicon, even among the general public, very quickly. People, including myself, would think: 'It's OK, because they had underlying health conditions. Oh, that's fine then. I don't have underlying health conditions. I'm OK.'

A couple of days would go by and we'd get another one:

'We've had our fourth death; they were in their 70s with underlying health conditions.'

After that, those emails suddenly stopped. A week went by and there were no reports of individual deaths. The next email we received was very different. It jumped to what we would then get for the next few months: an outline of the number of suspected and confirmed cases of coronavirus and the number of deaths. I'd guessed it was because the numbers of those afflicted by the virus were increasing rapidly and that telling employees about a young person dying would be a big blow to morale. That would have broken people. It certainly had an impact on our department, because in A&E we often follow our patients up to see how they have progressed after we have admitted them to the hospital. We can only get very limited information from the computer system; you can see what investigations they're having done or if they're due for discharge. Sometimes you see a pink hash mark over the name and that means they've died. It's always a shock when you see that. I don't know why it was always pink; red was perhaps too harsh, so they chose pink – a softer shade that wouldn't jump out at you and remind you of teacher's corrections on your homework. It didn't make it any less arresting when you saw it.

In the first months after I qualified as an ACP, I followed up every single patient I saw. I'd come in half an hour before my shift started and log on to the computer. It became part of my daily routine. My colleagues saw me doing it and would say, 'You need to stop that.' I ignored them, calmly doing my checks until one day I typed in the NHS number of one patient and the pink hash mark was across her name. 'What?' I thought. 'She was only in her fifties. How has she died?' I had admitted her to the gynaecological ward when she presented with lower abdominal pain. She seemed fine when I left her, and then she died. It was a horrible, gut-wrenching shock, followed by feelings of immense guilt and self-flagellation. What did I do wrong? What did I forget?

The dreaded pink hash mark is how we found out that a young patient had died of Covid-19. The patient was in their twenties and had been admitted to intensive care while I was on shift. They were normally fit and well, like me. The clinician who treated them would have looked them up to see how they were doing. That kind of bad news spread fast. When a second patient in their thirties died I suddenly knew I wasn't invincible.

The initial messaging around coronavirus only being fatal in the old and vulnerable was really harmful. It took my knowing about two patients who didn't fit that criteria for my husband and I to start treating this virus seriously. Before each shift he would start to say, 'Be careful,' with some sincerity. Normally he makes a joke about me going off to save lives. I always replied with a casual and breezy 'I'll be fine', but deep down I was bricking it.

I was on my way to work in the car one day not long after this when I had a horrible pain across the front of my chest. I was struggling to breathe. I was also getting palpitations. Oh God, was I developing coronavirus symptoms? I ran through what else might be wrong. It couldn't be a heart attack because I was in my early thirties. Could it be related to wearing PPE? It was difficult to breathe in, and so hot in the isolation unit. I put it down to that. The palpitations settled when I got to work but it continued to be an effort to breathe up to the point when I finished my shift. Then when I finished for the day and was out in the fresh air and not being tied down with extra equipment and clothing, I felt fine.

On my way into work the next day, the pain came back, only to disappear once again at the end of my shift. It became a regular pattern and I messaged a friend who worked with me saying that I didn't know whether I was coming down with something. Could it be the change in the weather? I'd go for a run and be absolutely fine. This was weird. What was it? I didn't understand. I couldn't be developing Covid-19 because none of my symptoms were getting worse. I didn't have a cough, either.

One night shift, a colleague came in after cycling to work and said that his chest was tight.

'Oh yeah, I've been getting that,' I replied. 'Maybe it's the weather?'

'Yeah, yeah, maybe,' he said.

It clicked a little while afterwards that these were probably physical manifestations of the anxiety I, and everyone else in the NHS, was facing. I had also felt this way after Dad died. I had never considered myself an anxious person or someone whose mental health took a knock. I always believed that exercise and fresh air could solve anything. My dogs were also an antidote to any stress I was feeling; when I had a rough day, looking into their doting eyes immediately made me feel better.

This entire year had been a test so far and cracks were beginning to appear in my own well-being. While I tried to swat away the thoughts that one of my colleagues, or I, might become victim to the virus, they crept in like dark clouds before a storm.

After lockdown had finally been announced, I felt a kind of relief, assuming people would really take this seriously now and stay at home. I was glad there would be no distractions like cafes, pubs and restaurants to tempt people out of their homes to mingle with others and the virus.

It soon became clear that some people were flouting the rules, however. Did they need to be told in exhaustive detail about the people my team saw who had so much life yet to live but who had been struck down by the virus? Some individuals seemed to think they were invincible. But it wasn't long ago that I had felt that way. I guess if you'd had no personal contact with the virus, it just seemed like a malevolent stranger in the corner, or on the other side of the road, who wasn't doing you any harm. It was still lingering there in the background though, ready to pounce at any given opportunity.

People would contact me telling me that they couldn't hack it anymore and that they were going to see their elderly parents, who I knew had health conditions that made them more vulnerable. I didn't really know what to say to them. Me and my NHS colleagues were ultimately the ones who would deal with any negative consequences of reckless action. I found myself getting increasingly annoyed with my glamorous neighbour; she was in her eighties (though she looked decades younger) and kept having friends and her boyfriend round to her house on a regular basis. I guess if I got to that age, maybe I wouldn't give a damn. Was it something about seizing every day and going out on a high? I was also a bit put out that I, and so many other healthcare professionals, were putting our lives at risk, and dying in some cases, while others were out and about seeing friends and family with no guilty conscience. It was a double whammy; not only was my work focused around treating this new virus, but I wasn't able to see my family either.

In the isolation unit, all the days seemed to merge into one. But each new shift saw new challenges and lives that had been touched by Covid-19. There was a stream of patients coming into the hospital and it wasn't always just the patient in front of me who was a victim of the virus, but also their families at home. There was the man who returned from work feeling unwell, then symptoms began a few days later for his elderly mother, resulting in her being hospitalized. Soon after, I saw his wife, who was sat in front of me, struggling with her breathing and not able to talk in full sentences, shaking with rigors as her temperature soared.

I saw one woman in her eighties who didn't understand why she was in A&E. As I assessed her, I felt uncomfortable because she had dentures that didn't fit properly and that kept clattering really loudly. It was off-putting. Enid was a lovely woman who normally resided in a care home.

'I feel unwell,' she kept saying.

'Is there anything more you can tell me about how you're feeling?'

'I feel unwell.'

'Can you be a bit more specific?'

'No, I just feel unwell.'

That was all she could tell me. Normally, a carer would be there to help shed light on the situation, but trust guidelines didn't allow any visitors into the hospital during the coronavirus outbreak. I phoned the care home who told me she had spiked a temperature. I did some investigations and they all pointed towards Covid-19. She also had a kidney injury and I thought it would be safer to admit her into hospital so we could keep a close eye on her.

For patients over the age of sixty-five, we automatically determine what clinical frailty score they have.

It's a scale of one to nine. One is the lowest, which is where a patient is completely independent, while nine is someone considered to be fully dependent on care and anticipated to die fairly soon. Each level has check-points so it's quite easy to determine where someone lies on the scale. Enid was a six. We had recently been told that if we were admitting someone with a score of six or seven, then we had to consider signing a DNAR form (Do Not Attempt Resuscitation).

I went back to tell her.

'Enid, we're going to bring you into hospital for a little bit,' I said. She suddenly came out with: 'I don't want resuscitating.' It took me a bit by surprise so I gathered myself and then we had a conversation where I learnt she was a retired doctor. She obviously knew best and had probably filled in loads of DNARs in her time.

It was a relief, if I'm honest. It meant I didn't have to broach the subject with her. Conversations with patients and/or relatives about death are really hard. It's not a pleasant chat to have, and death is still a taboo subject which people are scared to talk about. It's also so easy to be misunderstood as a healthcare professional. You want the best for your patient but often people will interpret you suggesting the possibility of completing a DNAR as giving up. That's not the case at all. We make every effort to make patients better; we give them fluids and antibiotics but if a frail ninety-three-year-old woman with various health problems goes into cardiac arrest, it's probably not in her best interest for us to start jumping up and down on her chest to bring her back. What would she be coming back to? Probably a vague semblance of a life where she had no independence and couldn't feed or toilet herself.

Sometimes relatives get angry and defensive. You have to be careful with the words you use and how you say them. 'If their heart was to stop, this is what we would do and she might end up in the intensive care unit with a tube down her throat. Would you want that for her?' Sometimes the answer is yes. We respect their wishes but my heart sinks when I hear this. It's cruel to resuscitate people sometimes and if family members witnessed the procedure, they would probably ask us to please stop. In that situation, I ask the wards where my patient is due to go to try and bring up the subject again. They often have more time than we do in A&E. It's such a sensitive topic that it can take a good hour to discuss it. Of course, we are beholden first and foremost to the person we are caring for and if we really believe that resuscitation would do more harm than good, we wouldn't do it. Our job is to do what is in the patient's best interests.

At this point, I hadn't had to deal with many elderly patients with Covid. I was grateful for this as conversations with families were only allowed over the phone, making the discussion of such a difficult subject even harder.

Later that shift I got a text message from Ed saying that he thought people at his work were beginning to get nervous because he was living with a healthcare professional. His office was still open and he had to go in two or three days a week. Someone must have said something to him. They got their money's worth out of me, though, when my health advice kept being quoted in management meetings. They bought thermometers for people to use because I'd told them that a temperature of 37.8 degrees or above suggested someone should self-isolate as it could be coronavirus.

Then, a couple of weeks later, Ed told me they were considering getting sats probes in so that people could monitor their oxygen levels. 'That's a terrible idea,' I said to him before going on to explain that medicine is not an exact science and that individuals' normal oxygen levels differed according to various factors, like whether they had certain respiratory conditions, for example. My husband sat with a pad taking notes before scurrying back into the study and dialling into a teleconference call. A while later he emerged and confirmed that they had decided not to get oxygen sats monitors. Was I going to get paid for this consultation work?

Like a lot of other people as March slipped into April, I wasn't sleeping properly. By this time, more than 5,000 people had died in UK hospitals and the accelerating US death toll was closing the gap with Italy and Spain, who had also been hit hard by the virus. I'd often spend hours lying awake past midnight mulling over the patients I had seen that day and replaying in my head everything I'd done. When I was asleep, I dreamt that I was at work. Even my sleep-talking was dominated by this new dystopian world I found myself in; one night I said, 'I find it all quite lonely,' while on another occasion I spoke about blood. The reason I know is because my talking woke my husband up and he wrote down what I said and sent it in a text message for me to read when I got up the following morning. For him, it was amusing. I, meanwhile, felt as though I never had a break and like I was at work twenty-four hours a day.

Time off at home with nothing to do was hard at times. When I had a moment to sit and think about what was going on around me, I felt terrified. I was hearing that my fellow health workers were dying. Some of our ambulance crews and bus drivers with the trust lost their lives to the virus. I hadn't treated them personally in A&E, but the news made us realize how very close to home the virus was. We had recently lost a valuable and loved member of our team, who had a ruptured brain aneurysm and that had a horrible impact on the workforce. We made a promise to be more like him – a loving, caring and joyful nurse who always brought a smile to everyone's faces, no matter what difficulty we were facing at work. I felt really vulnerable and would look around the department wondering if the person working near me might die. I had a lot of morbid thoughts, especially because I knew that corona-virus did not discriminate. Everyone was aware of the dangers and the entire hospital was worried, for them-selves and others.

I feared death, or worse – giving my husband the virus. The possibility was there. It wasn't something I could avoid. I didn't have a choice about going into work; it was my job. I had to care for those patients because it was what I was meant to do. I couldn't say no, or avoid them because I was fit and well. I couldn't keep two metres away; I couldn't not touch patients or avoid getting close to them when I needed to listen to their chest. I felt scared.

I took the dogs out a lot more and appreciated my time in nature with them. I tried to read novels and binge watch Netflix so that I had a break from the news or research papers about Covid-19. I tried to turn off but it didn't help when Ed would reel off the latest figures of people who had coronavirus and those who had died from it. He's always loved letting me know about the latest developments reported by the media but it got to the point where I didn't want to know anymore. 'I don't want to hear it,' I eventually told him and he stopped.

I didn't really know how he was feeling. He's not very good at showing how he feels and bottles things up a lot. He cried at our wedding so I knew he was capable of emotion, but he doesn't seem to express it well. He's a bit of a monotonous machine. Every now and then he would hint that he was worried, however. Communication has never been his strong point.

Ed's strength of character lay in his reliability and practicality. He was very capable and never let me down. I was never more glad of this than when I lost my car key on a run before a night shift. I'd finished at 8 a.m. that morning and had woken up at 11.30 a.m. desperate for the loo. It always happens that way, which is most annoying because I usually can't get much more sleep afterwards.

I decided to take the dogs out for a run down by the river. Halfway through, I realized my car key was no longer in my pocket. My house key and phone were in the car, which I had locked. I retraced my steps angrily. The grass was long and trying to find my car key was impossible. I continued along my original route and was hatching Plans B and C when I came across a mother and her two daughters who were out walking.

They initially looked shocked. I guess it's not every day that people are asked by a pink-faced, agitated woman with two dogs attached to her waist if she can use their phone. I had tried to look as honest as possible and not like someone who might run off with any prized belongings. Thankfully it worked and one of the daughters lent me her phone to call my husband. He was at work but his boss was forgiving and let him leave early to come and rescue me. I waited an hour for him to cycle home, pick up the spare car key and then cycle further to find me. I even managed to get an extra hour's nap in before my night shift.

My sister, who is single, would often say that it's hard not to have anyone to rely on who would drop everything to come to her aid. I was not particularly sympathetic when she brought it up but in that moment I got a glimpse into how our lives differed in that respect. I realized how much of a steady and reassuring presence Ed was in my life, now even more so than when my father was alive.

That night I was in the isolation unit, again. I decided to send a woman home who I strongly suspected had the virus. She was short of breath, had a fever and was coughing continuously. At that point we were only swabbing patients who were being admitted to hospital to find out definitely if they had coronavirus. I wished I could test more because the numbers about how widespread the virus was were not a true representation of what was really going on. And some people came in wanting to know for sure if they had contracted it. I had to send them home saying they probably did have it but we couldn't be certain.

We couldn't admit everyone to hospital and this woman would have been just as well off at home, where she'd be more comfortable than on a ward.

'I feel awful,' she said. 'Are you sure it's OK for me to go home?'

'I can absolutely sympathize with how dreadful

you're feeling, but there's no point in you staying here. We can't do anything more for you. You're just as well off being at home where it's more comfortable.'

I also knew I had to protect her and other patients so I gave her advice on what to do and told her that if her symptoms worsened to come back.

The terror in her eyes was palpable. She was scared to go home and she didn't trust her own judgement.

'How do I know when I'm unwell enough to come back?' she asked.

I didn't really know how to answer. She was going to continue to have a temperature, feel short of breath and have chest pain, which were all signs you needed to come to A&E normally. How could I explain to her how to recognize the point when the symptoms were so bad she should bring herself back to the emergency department? It was hard. I tried to reassure her as best I could but she was crying and shaking. People naturally get upset when they're unwell. I cry if I vomit because I hate it so much. Add a pandemic that was killing thousands of people around the world into the mix, and people had every right to be more worried. When the news was full of daily statistics stating that hundreds were dying each day, I couldn't blame people for being more anxious. All my suspected Covid-19 patients were this way. I tried to reassure them, but I didn't know how effective I was.

After she left, I heard the patient opposite tell someone: 'Careful, mate, you don't want to go that way,' as he pointed towards where my patient had been. 'She had the virus.'

Did he need reminding that he too was in the isolation unit and therefore also suspected of having the virus?

5

The Way It Should Be

As the weeks passed we waited nervously to be overwhelmed by cases, not knowing when the pandemic
would peak, still less when it would end. The cases
rose every day and our two isolation units in A&E
became three. There was one day in mid-April when
all three units were full and it looked like we'd need
a fourth. The number of deaths in England each day
was surpassing 1,000 with scary regularity. On the
whole, however, everything still felt manageable at
work, on a resources level. Preparations were thorough
and loads of money was injected into the NHS. It was
strange to experience this after working through several
winters where we were constantly under pressure with
no free beds in the hospital. It seemed to get worse
every year too.

During previous winters, emergency departments
would be overcrowded with patients waiting for a bed
to become available on the ward. Clinicians were
expected to review a patient's regular medications, make
sure second, third and fourth doses of antibiotics were

prescribed and re-review their patients. Nurses would be trying to keep up with the endless mixing and drawing up of intravenous medications in amongst making sure they turned patients every two hours to reduce the risk of pressure sores. Hot meals were being ordered in to try and cater for missed meal times. We were running a ward alongside A&E. Staff were demoralized.

There was one incident that really illustrated to me how winter pressures affected everything. During my training to be an ACP, I was supernumerary so wasn't included in the official numbers of people working in the department. All my work was supervised by a consultant. One shift, there was an unprecedented eight-hour wait to be seen by a clinician. The next patient on the list was a woman in her forties who had fallen off her bike. I felt I shouldn't be seeing her because she was a trauma patient and that was out of my remit. I spoke to the consultant and he was happy for me to go in and take an initial look.

When I entered the cubicle, the woman was grey, sweaty and agitated – never a good sign. Her abdomen was distended and rigid and she was writhing around in pain as the painkillers the nurses had given her were wearing off. Her observations had remained stable so far, but now she had low blood pressure and a high heart rate. She had ruptured her spleen when she'd hit her abdomen going over the handlebars, a common injury for cyclists.

She had been triaged correctly and was meant to have been seen within twenty minutes, but because the department was so busy with patients who all seemed to be needing immediate attention, that was just not possible. After I saw her, she was quickly sent round to resus and then taken to theatre. Had I not taken her on, she would have waited even longer and potentially have deteriorated. She was already at a tipping point and was bleeding internally.

There was such a stark contrast between pre-Covid and Covid days in our A&E, as there was for many departments across the country. For one thing, coronavirus brought healthcare professionals from different specialities flocking to our aid. Everybody was being so helpful and supportive. Before, I'd sometimes refer a patient and be met with resistance. One speciality would say it wasn't their problem, send them elsewhere; the other speciality would say the same. A&E would always be caught in the middle, arguing, and it shouldn't have been our responsibility. We'd go back and forth and it would delay our ability to see the next patient. What a waste of time over stupid politics.

When Covid-19 took over, referring a patient became a very smooth process. With elective surgeries cancelled, orthopaedic doctors would come and run our minor injuries units which were usually run by nurse practitioners. Patients were getting gold standard care. There were more consultants and more staffing in general. Staff who'd left A&E returned for a few months. We used to have four doctors on one shift before; now there'd be around twenty. Before, when we were in the thick of winter, patients could wait for over four hours to be seen; now I'd see them within ten minutes of arrival. I couldn't believe it.

When the pandemic struck and attendances to A&E dropped, patient flow through the hospital became a slick process. Patients weren't in A&E for a minute longer than they needed to be and nurses were able to give the care people deserved and left after their shift feeling content. It was one of the positives that came out of the crisis and what A&E should be like.

I woke up one morning and scrolled through my phone bleary eyed. Amid the posts about how everyone's lockdowns were going, the animal videos and memes, there was a message from my trust on their Facebook page. It read: 'Can you help us? Do you have any stock of new full-length coveralls that you can donate to us to help keep us safe?'

Were we running out of PPE? This was the last thing I wanted to hear before I went on shift later that day. I was aware that healthcare professionals all around the country were crying out to be kept as safe as possible at work. In the news, there had been pictures going around of nurses wearing bin bags in an attempt to protect their clothes. Some paramedics refused to go into houses to resuscitate people suspected of having coronavirus because they weren't kitted out with adequate PPE. This lack of essential equipment was adding to the strain of everyone working in the NHS. Not only that, but it soon emerged that the virus was ripping through care homes; people working there also needed PPE but weren't getting it.

Back when we were still working out what level of PPE we needed in different scenarios, everyone was very uneasy. UK guidelines differed from what the World Health Organization was recommending at one point. I went from not needing to wear anything, to being fully gowned from head to toe, to wearing a full coverall in a matter of weeks. There was a good period of time where advice was constantly changing and people were questioning things because they weren't sure what the latest guidelines were dictating. At one stage, the guidance changed twice in one day. As the virus was ramping up, so was our PPE.

Once, I gave a patient nebulizers (medications delivered through a mask that are used to help clear airways) without wearing full PPE but was told off by my consultant for not moving them into a separate room specifically designated for aerosol generating procedures. Weeks later, that procedure was still not listed in official guidance as an aerosol generating procedure so I had been right all along. I felt bad about being told off but perhaps it was for my protection. There were so many conflicting instructions. I just wanted to get to the point where we had to wear full PPE; this constant indecision felt risky and very frustrating.

Dozens of healthcare professionals had died by that time. One of the first to pass away was an ear, nose and throat surgeon. The nature of his job meant that he had to get close up to people's noses and mouths. Had he been wearing PPE? Did he need to die?

I was really angry because this seemed to be a massive failure for no logical reason. My brother-in-law in China was sending pictures of his school where everyone was wearing an excessive amount of PPE. When I was taking a break in the staffroom one shift, I watched a news programme where they interviewed the manager of a factory who had got in touch with the government to see if they needed him to make more PPE. They ignored him. He continued making it, but was sending it to other countries.

I thought about those less fortunate than myself. Luckily for me, there was only one occasion where I went for lunch and afterwards couldn't go back in to the isolation unit because there were no supplies of PPE left. Some was found but it was a good hour before I was allowed back in. On another occasion, I had been told to wipe down the PPE I was wearing so that it could be reused. Again, more supplies were found in time so I didn't end up having to do this.

I couldn't imagine what it would be like for those health and care workers without adequate PPE.

No one should be made to choose between helping another person and putting their own life and others' in danger. I could see early on that it would be a major feature in the daily routines of many of my wider colleagues. I was glad I had never been put in that position.

The ethics and morals surrounding Covid went further than that though. Difficult decisions were a recurring theme in healthcare. So far, I still hadn't had to make any during the pandemic that were particularly vexing. Either my patients were all previously fit and it was obvious that they needed to be given every possible treatment, or they were old and frail and already had a DNAR, wanted one, or it wouldn't have been fair to resuscitate them.

That didn't mean people weren't grappling with decisions up and down the country and abroad, however. I knew colleagues were facing difficult decisions every day. Those in A&E or on the wards were calling intensive care doctors to come and review their patients to see whether they were to be put on a ventilator. Some weeks before, they might have been accepted because there was room. But it was different now. Covid patients were sicker for longer, and many did not survive. Some units were getting full; professionals from other specialities were being drafted in to help and nurses were being stretched thin and having to look after more patients than normal. The data around who was more at risk was changing all the time, as were the parameters of who survived this new virus.

To some extent, these decisions were taking place all the time before Covid was a twinkle in a Chinese bat's eye. Each patient that came in to A&E and needed further treatment was an individual case and it was important to consider how far we should escalate them. Usually, the decision was made by the intensive care doctor. They'd come and review a patient and say, 'Let's give it a go, I think the patient has a good chance,' or, 'No, we're not going to take them.' For me, it was a relief that I didn't have to make these decisions; they were made for me. Those in intensive care are the ones who look after the patients; they know a lot more about how they would cope with being intubated. Time on the ICU involves a lot of really aggressive medications; it's a fine balance knowing if someone will tolerate that or not.

Although we didn't know much about the virus, we knew how it affected the body, the lungs and the impact it had on the rest of the organs. If there was a patient with a bad heart, you might not know the ins and outs of the virus, but you knew that the necessary medication would take a heavy toll on their heart. Their history would give you a clue as to how they might do on a ventilator.

Often, I'd be told that a patient was not suitable for intensive care. That didn't mean it was the end, though. We could escalate them to the high dependency unit, or they'd get ward-level care. We did everything we could and hoped that the patient rallied. Sometimes they did and that would be a pleasant surprise; sometimes they wouldn't and I'd think, 'We can't save everyone, maybe it was their time.'

Having to explain this to relatives was very tricky and fraught, however. Similar to when I had to bring up DNARs, they would jump to the conclusion we were leaving their loved one to die, that because they weren't going to intensive care, their relative was end-of-life. I'd explain this wasn't the case: intensive care wasn't always successful and it wasn't right for the patient in this situation; they would absolutely continue to receive the best care that the hospital could provide.

I'll always remember one patient who came in after she'd banged her head on a stone slab after falling over in the garden of the care home she was living in. I scanned her head and it showed she had a big bleed. I discussed it with the vascular surgeons and they said the chances of her surviving an operation were so slim, it wasn't worth putting her through it. She was to be admitted to a ward to be cared for and to see whether she might die or recover.

I was convinced these were her last moments of life. She was barely conscious. I thought she was dying in front of me. She took about four breaths a minute; she was gasping for air. I brought my consultant in and he reviewed her, agreed with my prognosis and we signed the DNAR form together. Then we went to talk to her two children.

'I don't think she's going to make it,' I told them. 'I can't predict how long it will be but we'll make sure she's comfortable. This is it, I'm really sorry. I think you should get all your relatives to come in so they can see her if they want to.'

They were in floods of tears. I didn't know then that four days later I would be proved wrong. I followed her up and she was sat on the ward, talking, eating, drinking and walking. She was due to be discharged back to her nursing home. I could not believe it. Some people are so hardcore and stoic; they seem to go on forever.

Week five of lockdown had arrived. This was how I was measuring time at this point. The days all blurred into one, and life had changed so dramatically that lockdown became a marker, a bit like the birth of Jesus. Wouldn't it be funny if that's how time was measured in the future, I thought? Instead of BC and AD, we'd use BL and AL.

Despite the restrictions on daily life, people were still getting themselves into trouble. I walked into one cubicle at work and was confronted by what I can only describe as a man who looked like a gangster. He had lots of gold teeth that reflected the harsh glow of the fluorescent lights. He was under arrest and had been brought in by the police.

I got down to examining him, or trying to. He was so rude. He had a fracture on his hand and it took several attempts to get an X-ray as he kept moving it. The radiographers refused twice to do it due to his behaviour. I had to act as the go-between, bridging political and social divides like I've had to do so many times before in my career in A&E.

'Bruv, but I'm in pain, yeah?!' he said to me when I tried for the third time to get him to cooperate.

'I can't do anything until I get this picture of your hand. Either you go home or you sit here for two minutes in a slightly uncomfortable position and have your hand X-rayed,' I told him sternly.

'All right, all right.'

The X-ray revealed he had broken his hand. We managed to get a cast on him and I was glad to pass his care to Orthopaedics, who'd call him the next day.

Pre-Covid, there wouldn't be a week go by without us seeing at least one person with a stab wound come into the department. It was even more prevalent before I started working in the hospital. Gangs are still around, however, and there are certain family names that are synonymous with gang culture. The situation reminds me of the bitter rivalry between the Montagues and Capulets in *Romeo and Juliet*. Every now and then, I'd treat a patient and an older member of staff would see their name and make comment. Now, those families have members behind bars and their drug-dealing operations seem to have been shut down – or else they are more underground.

Not long after I first started as a nurse, a senior colleague took me to one side to tell me about what had happened regarding gangs in the area. She told me a story about a man who had been badly beaten up and left in the car park outside the doors of the department. The people that were with him had brought him by car and pushed him out before they drove off. It was only because a member of staff had gone outside for a cigarette that they saw him and brought him in for treatment. The whole department then had to be sealed off because there were rumours that the rival gang wanted to come and finish him off. I wasn't sure how effective that would be as we have so many entrances; we're a vulnerable department. I couldn't stop thinking about the parallels with television dramas I'd seen over the years.

The stories of victims of gang crime are always opaque. They won't tell you how they got their injuries, or what happened or who did it to them. Police will appear and they'll be on first-name terms.

'Was it [insert name here] who did it to you?' the police will ask.

'Dunno, bruv,' the patient will reply. They can't rat someone out because that gets them into more trouble.

Knife crime is a major problem where I work and for the past couple of years we've had a group of social workers who we refer cases of gang violence to. They work with people under the age of twenty-five to try and prevent them from getting into gang life, or to get them out of it. They're amazing and some of them have their own gripping story to tell.

There was one case that shook the city and epitomized how sad and brutal gangs can be. One teenager had managed to escape a gang in another city; he'd been given a new name and was just starting out in a new life. He was known to safeguarding teams across the country, and to us since he'd come into A&E before. One night he was brought into A&E with such severe injuries that he died. His gang had caught up with him. We were all gutted because everyone had been so excited for his future after he'd left the gang. He'd been really difficult to work with at first but was showing promise. It just showed how hard it was to escape that life once you were embroiled in it.

One night we had three people with stab wounds in the department and two of them knew each other. They were shouting across to each other over the curtains.

'Is that you?' asked one.

'Ah, mate, how you doing? What are your injuries?' the other replied.

'Yeah, mate, they got me good.'

Their injuries were almost a badge of honour it seemed.

Once I spent four hours suturing seventeen stab wounds on a man. He had a couple of dangerous ones, but most were superficial and he didn't even need to go to theatre. On that occasion, he was under arrest and there was a police officer in with me.

'I'm going to suture your wounds,' I told him.

'What does "suture" mean?'

'You're going to get a load of stitches.'

'Oooooooh! How many stitches will I have?'

'I'm not sure yet, I'll have to see how I go. There are a fair few wounds so I'd imagine quite a few.'

'Alright, then.'

He seemed almost happy, like it was cool to have loads of stitches. I got to work and it wasn't long before the patient drifted off to sleep, so I ended up talking to the officer. Public service professionals often swap notes on how their shift is going. We all see ourselves as part of a big team of emergency services so there's a lot of camaraderie. We come across the same issues and characters, and receive a fair bit of abuse too.

Later on that shift my consultant approached me.

'Ah, Louise, mmmmmm, errrrrr . . .'

'Yeah?'

'I've ermmmmm, ermmmm . . .'

'Yeah?'

'Errrrrr, I've just got errrrrrr a bit of a favour, if that's OK?'

'Yeah?'

He went on to ask me to perform a rectal examination on his young, female patient.

'Better to have a woman do it,' he said.

I understood where he was coming from. It would be more appropriate for a female to perform the exam anyway. Rectal examinations are very awkward procedures that can be really traumatic for patients if they're mishandled. They are done to determine if there's any bleeding from the rectum, or if someone hasn't opened their bowels in a while to check the stool and what consistency it is. You have to feel how smooth the rectal wall is, or see if there are any tumours, or feel for the prostate in men and whether it's enlarged.

When I came off my bike as a student and ended up as a trauma patient in A&E, I had one myself. I was very drugged up when they turned me to do an assessment. We call it a log roll and it involves four people who turn you over while protecting your spine. No one told me what was going on; I felt people's hands all over me invading my personal space. One pair of hands goes between the thighs, close to your crotch. There's little dignity in it and every time I do it I always make sure I talk a patient through what is going on. It can be really triggering for a patient, particularly if they've been sexually abused.

It's also quite scary because you feel like you're going to fall. You can't move because you're strapped down to a spinal board and suddenly you're turned and all you can see is the floor. Next, someone feels down the spine and, in some cases, your anus to see if your ability to squeeze your bottom is still there. When I was a patient, though, they did it with no warning. All of a sudden I had someone's finger up my ass and my drug-induced stupor disappeared. I felt vulnerable and violated and I just wanted my mum and dad to be there with me.

It's one of those procedures that just needs to be done as quickly as possible, for everyone involved.

I went into the cubicle where the woman that my consultant had asked me to see lay in pain.

'Hello, my name's Louise. I'm here to do an examination in your back passage,' I said. Some of the medical terminology we healthcare professionals use is so alien and not common parlance so I always gauge facial expressions. Usually the reaction is one of horror accompanied by 'Oh God.' That's when I know the patient understands what needs to be done.

'Look, I know it's not very nice. Hopefully it won't be painful, just a bit uncomfortable and an odd sensation but it's over in a few seconds and it's really important that I do it,' I usually say.

Some patients have had them so many times before that they'll drop their trousers straight away without a word. Others sometimes refuse.

This woman was very obliging and thankfully the examination showed there was nothing to worry about and that she could go home.

I once had a patient who was a man only a few years older than I was. I explained that we needed to perform a rectal examination and was he OK with that. My consultant had come in to watch me because it was during my training and this made me feel more nervous than usual. I did it and when it was over the patient said, 'Don't tell my wife, but I quite enjoyed that.' I felt myself go bright red.

Another procedure that can be awkward for both professional and patient is catheterizing someone. A urinary catheter is usually used when people have difficulty peeing naturally. It can also be used to empty the bladder before or after surgery. When I qualified as a nurse, I was only allowed to insert catheters into women. I'm not sure why, because inserting them into men is usually a lot easier. I always found that rule really bizarre. Now I am allowed to do them on men and women.

A woman's anatomy varies from individual to individual and trying to find the urethra, where the catheter goes, can be quite difficult sometimes. It's not that uncommon for the catheter to be misguided up into the vagina in error. It's a very uncouth process; the patient lies flat on their back and spreads their legs. Then the healthcare professional has to delicately rummage around in their private parts.

One day during winter when the department was rammed full of people, I had to catheterize a woman with advanced dementia. It wasn't long before she shouted: 'Get your hands out of my fanny!' I was going as quickly as I could. I finished and opened the curtain to about fifty people staring at me. Luckily someone else was in there with me who could confirm that I was not molesting the patient.

With men it's much easier. There's a penis so you don't have to rummage because, generally, it's just there and you can hold on to it. There's only one hole and so not much room for confusion.

A couple of times, men have had erections when I've

been doing this. It doesn't bother me at all and I realize it's just a physical reaction to a sensitive area being touched.

I've seen hundreds of vaginas and penises, so many that I am always bewildered when popular culture and people are so obsessed with them. Both men and women can feel self-conscious about their private parts. These thoughts are often fuelled by popular culture, but everyone's unique. I've seen more vaginas than I've eaten chocolate biscuits, but as soon as I'm out of the room I've already forgotten what it looked like. I couldn't care less.

Penises on the other hand do sometimes leave an impression. The two largest ones I've seen belonged to two men, both aged a hundred. They were halfway down to their knees, absolutely humongous. I was in shock.

There have also been instances where there hasn't been a penis because it has receded so much. That can be quite a challenge when you need to help them go for a wee. There's nothing to put in the bottle so urine often goes everywhere. One time I had to push down on a man's abdomen and quickly grab what poked out. I don't really care and I don't know why they recede; sometimes there are medications that can cause it to do that. Nothing fazes me and I don't judge anyone. I'm there to do a job and that's it.

Some men get embarrassed, especially when a young, tall blonde comes in. I'm always very sensitive to any awkwardness and ask if they are happy for me to do it. I usually bring a chaperone too. Often they are really unwell and not in any fit state to give consent, or they're in urinary retention with two litres of liquid in their bladder. They're in so much pain because they can't pee so they don't care. They know that all I need to do is insert the catheter so the urine is released and then they're happy and grateful.

I've done hundreds of these types of procedures. I understand people can feel uncomfortable but they feel so much better when I'm done. They're also laid down flat, so looking at the ceiling and not me. Sometimes I'll make small talk to distract them, but sometimes I won't say anything at all.

At the weekend I decided to take advantage of the supermarket opening an hour earlier especially for NHS staff. I joined the queue and was stood there for fifteen minutes before I turned around to the woman behind me.

'Do you know why we aren't moving?' I asked.

'We're waiting for the NHS staff to have their time.' she replied. I hadn't realized that while I was able to start my weekly shop an hour before the general public, I had to go through a hidden back entrance to do so.

Going to the supermarket always reminded me of my parents. When I was growing up, Mum always said that if she was going to have a nervous breakdown, it would be in a supermarket. She would send Dad and my sister and me off to get certain products, and my sister would try and surreptitiously drop things that she wanted into the trolley without Mum noticing. When everyone was done, we'd all meet at the till and that's where the show began. My father would make a big scene, cracking countless jokes and asking for discounts. Sometimes he'd tell the person behind him in the queue that he'd forgotten his credit card and could he use theirs. He was like a minor celebrity at the local Tesco. Most of the time, people twigged that he was pulling their leg, but sometimes they wouldn't and it was left to my mum or me to smile and roll our eyes and say that he was joking. I found it really awkward when that happened. He wasn't bothered at all though, because he'd do the same every week, until he died.

As neighbours in the village and shopkeepers in the local town found out he had passed away, they'd share funny memories of him. The pharmacist told us they enjoyed his banter, the woman in the copy shop recalled him walking in and talking loudly about discounts and asking her to change the date on his digital watch because he didn't know how, and countless villagers recounted how he used to go and stand in the middle of the road and stop traffic at the crossroads first thing in the morning so that people could cross the road. As a deluge of condolence cards came through the letterbox, we opened them and 'character', 'larger than life' and 'kind' were some of the most common words and phrases people used to describe him. He would always be unforgettable to my mum, sister and me, but we soon realized that he had made an impact on more than us, and that was a comfort.

I felt the loss of my father even more keenly around the time of my birthday in late April. The daily number of lab-confirmed cases of coronavirus was the highest it had ever been and more than 4,000 were being recorded each day. In only one week there were thousands of people who died in the UK from Covid-19. I had the week off on annual leave; all previous plans to go to Pembrokeshire had been cancelled. It would have been wonderful; the weather that week was beautiful and I spent a lot of time in the garden. I tried an online yoga class outside but one of the dogs kept interrupting to lick my sweaty and salty face; the other one did a poo on the lawn.

That week, I woke up one morning to the news that a consultant in emergency medicine at a nearby hospital had died of Covid-19. Some of the consultants at the hospital I worked at had trained with him and were very upset. It further underlined that this crisis was very close to home and that no one was immune to it.

The same day we received our monthly payslip and it emerged that my colleagues had had a salary deduction due to the new pay deal that was brought in by the government. You had to laugh otherwise you'd cry.

My thirty-second birthday started with a pleasant surprise. I trundled down the stairs and into the kitchen where a five-tier rainbow cake with icing and unicorn confetti was sitting on the table. It looked so good that I automatically assumed my husband had bought it for me from the shop. He was standing looking very smug and proud of himself before he announced that he had made it in the middle of the night.

'Ha ha. Thank you, it's lovely. Where did you get it from?' I asked.

'I made it!' he replied.

'Come on. I know you didn't.'

'I did!'

We went back and forth for what seemed like ages before I started to get angry. I was tired of his joke, that wasn't funny anymore. I decided it wasn't worth arguing over and started getting my breakfast ready in a huff. As I put the empty milk carton in the bin, I saw evidence of Ed's late night cake-making session. He really had made it, and it tasted great too!

That wasn't the only rainbow I saw that day. The rainbow had become a symbol of support for key workers during the pandemic, which was why my husband had chosen to recreate it in cake form. As a wedding present, my cousin had re-vamped one of my grandpa's old wooden skis which was engraved with his initials and turned it into a shot stick. When it's not being used as part of a party drinking game, it takes pride of place on the living room wall. That morning, there was a rainbow caused by a diffraction of light resting on the ski. I took it as a supportive sign from beyond the grave. Either that or Grandpa was sending encouragement to start drinking shots at 8 a.m.

A birthday card had arrived from Mum. It was signed off 'love Mum', a sad reminder that this was my first birthday without Dad. He would normally have had a story to tell around my birth; most of the time it was that I arrived just in time for afternoon tea. I felt a pang of sadness at his absence. The card from my sister had a picture of an orangutan on it. It was meant to be me, she explained inside.

The next day I messaged my sister to ask for my godmother's number. It had been a while since I'd spoken to her. She gave me the news that my godmother had tested positive for Covid-19. She was eighty-nine and living in a London care home. News of care homes being ravaged by the virus was everywhere. She also had really bad asthma. She was part of the vulnerable group of high-risk people, but miraculously so far she was symptom-free.

'She's being taken to hospital,' my sister told me.

'What?! That would be a disaster. Why?'

'I don't know, that's just what she's told us.'

Not only would it cause distress by placing her in an unfamiliar and frightening environment, but it would also increase the risk of spreading the virus to the ambulance crew, the hospital staff and other patients. Hospitals are full of other bugs too; I knew the reality and it left me feeling infuriated and very pessimistic.

6

The Hidden Cost

I got home one morning after another tiring shift and noticed my elderly next door neighbour had a visitor pop round *again*. It felt like a direct affront to my work and it was annoying. Conversely, my other neighbour had dropped round a card and flowers saying thank you for all the work I was doing treating coronavirus patients.

There wasn't much time for my anger to simmer and possibly boil over as the next day I was back at work. I was in the minor illness section and relieved not to have to wear full PPE. That day I saw more people who shouldn't have risked coming into the hospital in the middle of a pandemic. I had to examine two pairs of breasts. This was not common practice in A&E as it's usually a complaint people go to their GP with. I wondered if perhaps people thought that their GP surgery was closed, or only offering tele-phone appointments, when they felt they needed to see someone face-to-face. They might have thought A&E was the only place they could see a healthcare professional in the flesh to get a problem checked out.

It was the end of April and the UK death toll had passed 26,000. I'd noticed on my way into work that the roads were busier and on my run there were a lot of people out and about. What were people doing? We were still in lockdown and there were hundreds of deaths from coronavirus each day.

In the next cubicle, a man was brought in because he'd snorted what he told me was a 'white substance' and wasn't happy about the effects it had had on him. He was under arrest and sharing his Covid conspiracy theories with the police; according to him, it was man-made and a bat was injected with it.

'What have you taken?' I asked him, needing more than 'white substance'.

'I don't know,' he said.

'It's important I know what you've taken,' I said. 'I can't really help you otherwise.'

Try as I might, he wouldn't give me any helpful information but there didn't seem to be anything seriously wrong. As I went to call my next patient in, he'd started on the Twin Towers and was explaining to the long-suffering policeman how it wasn't a terrorist attack that led to their destruction.

As I called my next patient in, the look of worry on her face and the fact she was clutching her abdomen told me almost everything I needed to know. She was pregnant and had been bleeding for some weeks. It had recently got worse and now she had a pain in her abdomen.

'Bleeding can be normal in the first trimester,' I said but tears quickly filled her eyes. I got a sinking feeling but told her to pop by the gynaecological ward to see if they could examine her. I saw her before I went home and she confirmed what we were both dreading: a miscarriage.

Miscarriages are painful, both physically and emotionally. It's a loss; a woman was expecting a baby and then she lost it. They can blame themselves and think they did something wrong but that is rarely the case. Sometimes they fear never being able to have children, and that is terrible.

I finished at midnight and drove home. Ed barely stirred as I got into bed. He was breathing heavily next to me as I lay there unable to sleep for a couple of hours as the day kept running over and over in my head. In the end I mindlessly watched a load of the cake-decorating videos that now filled my social media feeds. They were therapeutic and eventually sent me off to sleep.

The next day I was down to work in the isolation unit but there were no new patients to be seen. The consultant told me to wait outside to be called in if I was needed. He was trying to reduce the amount of staff who needed to put on PPE. I went to gulp down water in anticipation that it might be my only drink for hours. In the meantime, there were more patients to be seen in minors. Was this a good sign? Were Covid cases attending the hospital on the decrease?

That thought didn't linger long as my first patient told me she had lost the sense of taste on the left side of her tongue. Alarm bells rang as I knew loss of taste was a symptom of coronavirus. She had nothing else wrong with her, however, so I continued to take a history and went on to examine her. She was wearing a hat and a face mask which I asked her to remove so I could look everything over. She took them off and I saw a subtle droop on the left hand side of her face.

'Does your face feel normal?' I asked her.

'No, it feels like it's not working and when I drink, water dribbles out.'

This time, alarm bells rang for something else. I thought she was having a stroke. A stroke can be a life-threatening condition. It is a medical emergency and urgent treatment is essential. The sooner a person receives treatment, the less damage is likely to happen. 'Time is brain' is something we say. I was so thankful that I got to see her when I did, otherwise the situation could have deteriorated very significantly and quickly.

My next patient was a woman in her sixties. I checked to see what her presenting complaint was on the computer. I always like to get a bit of a heads-up so I know what I might be dealing with before I go and meet the patient. Managing expectations, I've learnt, is a big part of my job. It said: 'neck pain'. This could be one hundred and one different things and I ran through them all before I drew open the curtain to her cubicle. She could have twisted her neck getting out of bed in the morning; she could have had a carotid dissection, which is a tear in the inner layer of the wall of an artery; or she could have fractured her neck by falling off a bike perhaps.

I walked in and she was tearful. I hardly had time to ask why before she confessed, 'My partner tried to strangle me and it's not the first time it has happened.'

'OK, my name is Louise and the first thing I'm going to do is examine you to see how I can help. Is that OK?' She nodded but when I moved towards her, she winced. Her injuries weren't too serious so she was able to go home. But was home safe right now? She seemed to think so, but I was worried. I referred her to the domestic abuse team who would speak to her in more detail about her options and the possibility of finding a space in a refuge.

Up until that week, A&E had been quieter than usual. All over the country, hospitals and other NHS services were getting worried about people letting medical conditions get worse for fear of coming to hospital where the virus was rife. There were also fears that domestic abuse was on the rise, exacerbated by the lockdown. Calls to helplines had increased significantly and having come across patients suffering from domestic violence before, I could only imagine what was going on behind closed doors.

This was the second case of abuse I'd seen in close

succession. A few days before, we'd had to admit a woman who had been sexually exploited by a pimp for years. She was a victim of modern slavery and had escaped her own country where she had been tortured only to find herself working as a prostitute to pay back the money she owed her traffickers. She had turned up at A&E after managing to escape because she didn't know where else to go. There was nothing wrong with her medically, but she was referred to the safeguarding team who couldn't find a bed in a refuge for her for four days. We gave her a bed on one of the wards in the meantime.

Before Covid, people would attend A&E with a cover story for the injury that had brought them through our doors. Some came in repeatedly with abdominal pain, for example, and it can be hard for healthcare professionals to spot what's really going on. It's important to think outside the box, why does someone keep coming in? Are they looking for morphine because they're hooked on it, or are they trying to escape an abusive relationship at home? They come in to get away from the perpetrator. Then, there have been occasions where the aggressor is there with them and so it's even harder to determine whether they are being abused because they're so terrified they don't hint at what's really going on.

There have been times when I've asked someone directly, 'Is everything OK at home? Is someone hurting you?' and it's resulted in an outpouring of pent-up emotion and relief that they can finally talk about it. They'll open up, a whole can of worms erupts and I'm left speechless and horrified.

Other times, even when their injury doesn't match with their story, people will completely deny anything is going on. I've been working in A&E for eight years; I know what situations and accidents cause which injuries, and so do my colleagues.

One case that always sticks in my mind was a woman in her early twenties who said she had hurt her leg jumping down off a fence she'd had to climb over because a gate was locked. Normally when you jump off something, you get a certain type of fracture, or your ankle or knee might give way underneath you. Her injury was consistent with a blunt force against her leg which had resulted in the bone snapping. She was adamant she had jumped off the fence, however.

'Are you sure?' I asked her. 'It's very difficult to get your type of injury from jumping down from a height.'

'Yes.'

We have to go with what the patient says, even if the whole situation is dodgy. It wasn't long before her boyfriend came in. He was a great big hulk of a man and a fair bit older than her.

'Where's my girlfriend?' he asked before he found her and then wouldn't leave her side. He refused, even when we suggested it. To me, that confirmed something was going on. His behaviour was vile but she was so adoring of him.

'I love you, babe,' she kept saying.

The way he spoke to her was awful. 'What have you done now?'

'Babe, I'm sorry. I love you.'

Then he turned to me and asked: 'What are you doing to her?'

I replied, 'Do you mind giving us a few minutes of privacy please?'

'No I'm not going to do that. You don't want me to go, do you, babe?' he said, turning to his girlfriend.

'No, it's fine, he can stay,' she said.

'Sorry. I need to do something private and intimate. For this type of procedure I always ask that everyone leave for a bit so the patient can maintain a bit of dignity. I'll just be a couple of minutes,' I said while ushering him out of the cubicle.

'All right, but I'm just outside,' he replied.

At last I had a moment with her to myself. I asked if everything was OK at home and if he was being violent with her.

She denied it. 'I'm happy in my relationship,' she said.

'So what are these bruises all over your body?' I asked.

'Oh, I'm just really clumsy, I'm so silly.'

I had a gut instinct that all was not as it seemed and that something was very wrong.

It wasn't long before she was to be transferred up to a ward ready to go into theatre. I told the nurses that her story didn't fit her injuries. I said she had fingerprint bruises all over her body and could they try and speak to her again?

'You'll be a fresh face. I hope you have more luck than me,' I said to my colleague over the phone.

I let the safeguarding team in the hospital know too. We don't need a patient's consent for that when their safety is a matter of concern. They would look into the history, but now it was out of my hands. Our time with people is brief in A&E; we try to get the ball rolling and then pass it on to someone else.

I've seen a lot of patients in my career come in to the emergency department with wrist or facial injuries. They'll often say they walked into an open cupboard door. 'I'm really clumsy,' is a common phrase in this scenario. Sometimes they will be shaky and very timid. I'll look back at their records, and see they've been through our doors ten times or more over the past couple of years. There's clumsy, and then there's domestic abuse. Other times they will come in and say outright that someone has done it to them.

So many of the women I see in these circumstances go back to their partner. Domestic abuse charities say it can take an average of seven attempts to leave an abusive relationship. I always say, 'You don't deserve this, you don't need to go back.' It usually falls on deaf ears. 'He didn't mean it,' they usually say. It's so hard. I have to try and suppress my frustration.

I think about the person in front of me and wonder

what it is that leads them to go back. Why are they continuing with this relationship? Why don't they step away? To me, it's so straightforward. Someone hits you. Bam. You go, leave. Zero tolerance. I know, however, that there is an undercurrent of power and manipulation that stops victims from being able to escape.

I also then think, 'Hang on a minute, we've got zero tolerance to violence and abuse here in A&E.' And yet I've lost count of the number of times someone has been violent to me and I've continued to care for them. What I should really do is refuse. 'No. You've hit a member of staff. You should be arrested and leave the department.' Instead, I just carry on and make excuses. It's OK, because they're upset or drunk. Some victims of domestic violence I've met make excuses for their partner – they've had a bad day at work, they're stressed, I didn't clean the house properly.

I see far more female victims than male ones. I could count the number of male victims on one hand. I appreciate this probably isn't a true reflection of the number of male victims of domestic violence and that many of both sexes suffer in silence. I've also learnt that it's not just physical violence that constitutes abuse. Along with hitting, punching, using weapons, cricket bats and more, there's emotional abuse, financial abuse and controlling behaviour. I see it a lot and it has an impact on mental health.

From where I am in A&E, I see the devastation wreaked by years of funding cuts to refuges and domestic abuse services. There's not enough support. I think that's why so many turn up on our doorstep. We're seen as a safe haven. We're not really, but sometimes victims can't even look up a number for help on their phone because the aggressor controls everything. They can't leave the house unattended, or at all. So how do they get help? They come to A&E and feign a problem. If staff aren't clued up, we can miss it, tell them to go home and then that's it. They've lost their opportunity to get help.

I knew that lockdown most definitely was having an impact. Before, the perpetrator would have gone out to work for at least eight hours a day. Now, people were more frustrated, tensions were high, people's alcohol consumption had shot through the roof, making them more violent. Any crying children at home would have exacerbated the situation further. I couldn't escape news reports stating that calls to domestic abuse helplines had increased significantly, either. That was just those who were free and able to make the call. What about those who couldn't?

I went in the following day for the night shift and took handover for ten patients. I made a list of priorities and identified two patients who could be discharged home quickly. A win for them, and for me and the department. It was 10.30 p.m. Who wouldn't want to be in their own bed at this time? I knew that was what I was dreaming of.

Before I could make my way to the first patient to

discharge, I was stopped by a disgruntled woman. She didn't let me get a word in for a good five minutes while she complained about this, that and everything else.

'I've waited so long,' she started. 'This just isn't good enough.'

It's at times like these that I have to bite my tongue and remain passive and attentive. I've practised this skill to perfection over the years and it's stood me in good stead. I often think how lucky I am to have my temperament. I never heard my father raise his voice in anger, but my mother could get quite irate on occasion and my sister has a fierce temper, getting irrationally angry very quickly, and over nothing. So I listened calmly, thinking that if this patient would only let me talk, she'd find out that she was second on my list to discharge home. The only reason she wasn't first was because the other patient was elderly and I thought it fair to get to him first.

The disgruntled woman was no happier when I got to her but I quickly determined she was safe to go home. I told her, expecting relief, delight, or maybe even gratitude. Instead, she demanded to be kept in overnight. I was confused. I was also tired and wondered how far into my night shift I was. I glanced at my watch and saw I'd only been here for forty-eight minutes. I tried to understand why she was put out; she thought she'd broken a bone but nothing had shown up on the X-ray. Apparently, this had happened before though, and it had been missed and she'd been sent home before she'd had to be readmitted.

'I want to see someone more senior,' she declared.

'The consultant radiologist has reviewed your X-ray. You can't get higher than them,' I replied.

'Well, I can't go home because I'm living with people who have health problems and are vulnerable. What if I pass coronavirus on to them?'

I could understand why she was feeling anxious and it was a difficult time, but everybody had their own problems and situations that were highlighted by the crisis. At this point, the official global death toll had passed 225,000 and in the UK there were still around 800 deaths happening a day.

All I could think was, why would anyone want to stay in a hospital any longer than absolutely necessary during a pandemic? It would be the last place I would choose to be, except for the fact I worked there.

'I've got no way of getting home,' she went on to say. 'I was brought in by ambulance and it's your responsibility to make sure I get home safely,' she added. It never fails to amaze me how much I hear this. She was young, in full-time employment, fit and well. Why was a taxi out of the question? It turned out she was so reluctant to leave A&E because she was scared that her condition would deteriorate and there wouldn't be a medical professional immediately on hand to help.

I spent so long talking to her, going round in circles, aware of all the other patients still waiting. In the end

I had to leave her with my nurse colleagues, hoping they would have more success. A lot of patients seem to think the health service is a money tree, and there for people's convenience. It reminded me of stories I have heard from paramedics about people telling them not to block their driveway when parking before rushing into someone's house to perform life-saving treatment.

Midnight struck and heralded in a new day – the birthday of one of the nurses in my team. I drew her a happy birthday message adorned with balloons and fireworks on a napkin. Everyone signed it. It wasn't an elaborate card, but it was the thought that counted. I knew my A* in GCSE art would always come in handy.

The rest of the shift was uneventful. I hate it when the department is calm. Working nights is a trial in itself and not having much to do makes it that much harder. There's usually a definite rhythm; you start off feeling tired because it's bedtime and normally you'd be going to sleep. Then when you get into the swing of work and seeing patients, you perk up for a few hours. The lights are always on in A&E and it's loud whatever time of day it is. On the wards, the lights are dimmed so that patients can get some sleep. I find I'm usually OK until 4 a.m. when I start to feel sick and my vision tends to go a bit blurry. I can't wear my glasses when not treating coronavirus patients because the surgical mask I wear isn't tightly fitted and so the lenses would fog up. I get, what I have affectionately termed, night belly, where I get so bloated, it's uncomfortable. Normally, people pass wind when they're asleep but I can't do that when I'm working unfortunately; I don't think it would go down well with the patients.

I try to delay going to have something to eat for as long as possible because as soon as I do, I get sleepy. I try to eat at 5 a.m. because if I go for my break then, I know when I get back I've only got a few hours left, which translates to a couple of patients before hometime and my bed. The last hour of the shift is a slow crawl to the finish line. Everything hurts, my eyes get heavy, I still feel sick and I'm counting the minutes before those on the day shift arrive. Either that, or there's a rush of patients at 6 a.m., just as people wake up and discover something's wrong or that their problem which seemed like nothing to worry about has deteriorated overnight. When the new team come in all chirpy and fresh faced and take ten minutes to log on, I sit there wanting to scream at them to hurry up. It's worse when people try to make conversation with me at that time; by then I'm almost past the point of being able to talk. Forming words and coherent sentences is usually beyond me.

When it's busy, adrenalin keeps me going but it's so hard when it's quiet. On one recent shift I had looked through the drawers to see what advice leaflets were needed so I could go and print some off. I was so desperate to keep myself busy so I could stay awake that I'd do anything. I'd already cleaned everywhere and there were no patients to see. I never sit down because I would fall asleep and then that would be game over in terms of waking up again and carrying on. So, whenever I had nothing clinical to do I would walk, clean, re-stock and do anything I could find. After an hour, we got a flurry of patients. It's a bit like London buses, none come for a while and then a few come all at once.

When I got home, in my zombie-like state, I left the door of the kitchen open. The dogs usually have a morning walk with Ed and then stay in the kitchen behind closed doors when I'm sleeping after a night shift, otherwise I don't get enough rest. When we've left the door open before overnight by mistake, I get woken up by one of them whining and wagging her tail incessantly in anticipation of breakfast from around 4 a.m., or the sound of the other one's nails as he paces the wooden floors to find and get into the perfect comfortable position. I love them, but sometimes they drive me crazy. I woke up a few hours later to find them both lying as close as they possibly could on either side of my legs. We have a king-size bed but they chose those spots right next to me. I'd had three hours' sleep. I crawled to the bathroom, eyes still swollen shut, but it's so familiar that I don't need to be fully alert. I can find my way even when asleep. One of the dogs sat and watched me on the loo. I felt hungover for the rest of the day. Working nights is a double whammy.

You feel awful the next day and don't even have the joy and fun of a good night out to think about.

One of our regulars was in again. I was working in majors for my second night shift in a row. Bertha knew all of us by name, except she called me Lola instead of Louise. I hadn't corrected her. I saw her in town once where she approached me while I was doing some shopping. I'm sure I saw her more often than I did my husband. She'd been in and out of mental health services; she was sectioned for a while and I didn't see her for a couple of years. It had been a good amount of time since she had reappeared, though, and after a few weeks' absence because of Covid-19, she was coming into A&E on an almost daily basis. She had been in so often over the years that trying to find a vein for a cannula was nigh on impossible. Each time the location got more obscure. Today it was in her armpit.

Over my career in A&E so far, I've come across a number of people who come in regularly, hence the term 'regular'. Some have died, which is really sad; they had become part of the fabric of the department and I'd got so used to seeing them around. There were others who used to come in a lot who I hadn't seen in a while. Maybe they had all died, or maybe some had got the help they needed and got their life back on track.

One woman used to take massive overdoses, come

in, get minimal treatment and then abscond. She'd always be back a couple of weeks later. There was a man whose deep, booming voice meant you'd hear him before you saw him. He was an alcoholic and he died, as did the woman. Every time they came in, I'd take their bloods and wonder how they were still alive, because the results were not far off those of a dead person. I'd think, 'They're not going to survive this,' but then they would come back in the next time and I'd say to myself, 'Wow, they're still going.' I began to think they were invincible.

These people are from all walks of life and from a range of social backgrounds. I remember one woman whose father was rich and who kept giving her money to push her away. That just made feeding her drinking habit easier. She was difficult to work with. Once, she pissed on my foot. I'd run to get the commode, came back with it and placed it beside her. She got off the bed, lowered her trousers and squatted directly over my shoe before relieving herself. One time, she did a poo in the middle of majors and shuffled along leaving a trail of excrement behind her.

When I found out that one of our regulars had died I would have mixed feelings. There was an overwhelming feeling of sadness, but also of compassion. They had such tough lives; maybe they were at peace and no longer coexisting with the demons that haunted them while they were alive.

A small number of people had already started coming

back to A&E in early May with conditions that weren't Covid-related, and so had the regulars. 'I don't fucking care about Covid,' they'd exclaim. The ones I was dealing with at the time had such complex needs and were very challenging to manage. I had a couple of cases where people were in terrible pain but I couldn't find anything physically or medically wrong with them. I'd do every exam I could and all their results would be normal. They'd scream so loudly that it sounded like I was murdering them, and my colleagues would make jokes, warning me not to kill my patient. I was sure the problems were psychological and neither I nor the department were equipped to really help in these situations.

I always say to these patients that A&E is not the right place for them. I mean it in a supportive way. We can't do everything but people sometimes don't under-stand so get really upset. For someone with mental health problems, especially undiagnosed ones, the first step is to go to the GP. But they only have ten minutes for an appointment and for someone suffering from poor mental health, that's not enough. Maybe they'll be given some antidepressants but for someone who has experi-enced serious trauma, again that might not be enough. If they're lucky, they will be referred on to counselling, but even then the waiting list is months long. When someone is at a really low point in life, the last thing they think they can do is go on for months until they can talk to someone for one hour a week. Many understandably end up in A&E. Our brilliant mental health team is on hand in the department and we are considered a safe place by the police, but it's a nightmare. From our point of view, we like to rule out anything sinister that is immediately going to kill someone like a heart attack or a blood clot on the lung. Instead, more often than not, we see the sharp end of society's failings in dealing with mental health and the effects of years of underinvestment in services.

By this point of lockdown, I'd started seeing a massive influx in patients with mental health problems who had never had them before. When I'd seen the supermarket delivery driver weeks earlier I'd predicted that this would be an issue and I was right. One woman in her twenties had nothing physically wrong with her that I could find. She had come into A&E complaining of chest pain, but there was no clear medical cause.

'You're ready to go home,' I told her, before she burst into tears. Normally people are relieved that they're not at death's door.

'What's wrong? Is everything OK at home? Is someone hurting you?'

'No, no,' she replied. 'Everything's fine at home. My parents are lovely and so supportive. I don't know what's wrong with me but I feel terrible.'

'Do you think it might be related to your mental health? How do you feel you're managing at the moment?'

She looked at me so I continued, 'It seems to me

that you're low and perhaps struggling with a few things. That is having an impact on your mental health and now causing you physical symptoms such as this chest pain.' She nodded in agreement. 'You can book an appointment with your GP and they can refer you for ongoing support.' As I said this, I knew not all GPs were open, however. Some were doing telephone appointments. It was a disaster. People weren't able to be seen or get help so more were turning up at A&E with problems we couldn't treat. As she left to go home, I wrote a letter to her GP asking for a review and suggested referring her to a counselling service.

I went into another cubicle and was faced with a man pacing frantically; he was having an anxiety attack. He hadn't slept for three days and he was hyperventilating. He couldn't sit down, so his legs were hurting from not having any rest for days. I was getting tired trying to maintain eye contact with him.

'I am terrified of getting coronavirus,' he kept saying.

He was a supermarket worker and couldn't explain specifically what it was about coronavirus that was scaring him.

'I know I don't have it as bad as you working here in A&E,' he said. 'I'm sorry, but I don't know what I can do. I can't sleep, I can't function. I need help.'

He was shaking. 'I can't feel my hands,' he added.

'That's because you're hyperventilating. There's a build-up of CO_2. If you keep going on like this, you'll pass out,' I said.

I began to breathe with him, got him to slow down and we practised grounding techniques: breathe in for three, hold for four, breathe out for five with feet flat on the ground. After a couple of minutes he was managing to sit still and I began to talk to him and examine him to make sure this episode was anxiety and nothing else. I then went to speak to our mental health team and they said there was no need to admit him but suggested trialling him on a low dose of diazepam. When I went back he was fast asleep. I gently woke him up.

'Let's get you home. You can get some sleep and you'll feel so much better in the morning,' I told him.

'Thank you so much, you've really helped me,' he replied gratefully.

It felt amazing that I'd been able to help. He had completely transformed.

Covid-19 was having a colossal impact on mental health. Everybody was mentioning it. I was beginning to see a lot of people with chest pain. It is a common presentation in A&E but these people were in minors. They were young, in their thirties, and so were unlikely to be having a heart attack. I also knew I had experienced the same thing. I would say: 'I'm going to rule out a heart attack and anything else that might be life-threatening.' I'd eliminate everything and the only thing it could be was anxiety. I'd add: 'I've been seeing a lot more symptoms related to anxiety and I think the general public is underestimating the impact the virus has had on people.' Everyone was carrying on and insisting they were fine, but they weren't. It was affecting people without them realizing it. I'd explain that I did as much as I could to protect my well-being – going out into nature, exercising, eating well – but when I told them my thoughts, they'd agree. 'Yeah, it is affecting people.' Why wouldn't it? The lockdown was stressful and people were worried about isolation, job insecurity, relationships. Some had grief added into the mix.

Around the same time I saw four patients in one day who had tried to take their own lives. That was a lot for one person in one shift. It brought home to me how mental health isn't like physical health. People with physical ailments were mostly delaying coming in to the hospital because they feared catching coronavirus. People with serious mental health problems were in their own world of distress. When someone is in that state, they can't think about other things. Mental health problems couldn't be delayed until after the crisis was over; people didn't have the ability to escape from their dark thoughts.

My colleagues weren't immune either. I could see the worsening toll on their mental health too. People would say: 'I'm so over this, I've had enough.' One of my nurse colleagues who was hard as nails and had worked in A&E for years admitted that she had broken down in tears though she never normally cried. Loads of members of staff had had to move out of their homes and away from their families because they were so scared of bringing Covid home. I had never really entertained the thought of moving out of my house and away from my husband. He was young, fit and healthy with no underlying health conditions and so was low-risk, but I also knew I would have been lonely on my own and I needed his support. We also had two dogs to look after and he was working, not always from home. His company had started making parts for ventilators that the UK so desperately needed to treat those most affected by Covid-19. I loved that everyone came together and lent their skills to help. It also made me feel that we were all in it together, somehow. Although, I knew from what I'd seen in my job that not everyone was affected in the same way and that life most definitely was not fair.

The impact on those people who did move away from home was tremendous. Others kept telling me they had suddenly started crying and they didn't know why. Children were at home all the time. Staff had no time to themselves; one said she couldn't even go to the toilet alone. Everyone knew we would keep going but I was worried. In the winter, when we're usually at our busiest with skyrocketing pressure, people would hit burnout. And then what would happen?

Burnout has always loomed large over my career. It seems inevitable and I've always wondered how I'm going to survive until retirement age working in A&E. If I'm not at work, I am thinking about work. In the early days of my nursing career, I felt there was a fundamental insufficiency in mental health support for healthcare staff. With the increasing risk of burnout, we were putting ourselves, our patients and the profession as a whole at risk. It was important that I – and so many others – tried to remember that I was only human, while accepting that I work in a stressful environment. It wasn't going to get any easier, so I would just do what I could. That's all anyone could ask.

The trust was aware of the added burden on staff. They sent out a daily email with well-being tips. There was a room where you could go for biscuits, coffee and a sympathetic ear. Two prayer rooms had been set up for Ramadan for the first time. There were loads of posters on the doors in the bathroom talking about what to do at the end of a shift to decompress.

I was exhausted too. My work schedule was gruelling. I was working the large majority of unsociable hours and I didn't know how long I could keep going on like this. I had almost cried when I had a disagreement with a colleague. He had got angry with me for doing something that I knew I was right to do. I pulled him up on it and he later apologized to me. Others told me he had been off with them too. People were getting fraught and it was affecting some working relationships.

After my disagreement, I moved on to my next patient. He had been doing the washing up when he cut his hand on a broken wine glass. 'Why don't you have a picture of yourself stuck on your apron like I've seen on the news?' he asked.

'We're not in the Covid area of the department. Here we treat patients who aren't suspected of having the virus and so I don't need to wear full PPE,' I told him.

'You're quiet tonight, aren't you?' he went on to say.

A feeling of dread spread throughout my body. The word 'quiet' is banned in A&E. I'm not superstitious but everyone knows it's a jinx to utter that word at work. Whenever someone says it, it's not long until all hell breaks out. It's almost the equivalent of saying 'Macbeth' in a theatre. You don't mention the name; it's meant to bring bad luck. I know this because my mother was a professionally trained actor and spent some years on tour as well as working in Bristol and London, before she dramatically changed tack and moved out to the Sultanate of Oman to teach English, where she met my father. That wasn't the only knowledge my mother had imparted to me. She now worked as a counsellor and some of her clients had severe and enduring mental health problems, many of which were brought on by childhood abuse. I felt I had a deeper understanding of mental health issues and their origins because of her.

There have been times when someone's commented on it being quiet and then the red phone in resuscitation, alerting us to emergencies such as motorway pile-ups, where people have been seriously injured, has gone off seven times in the space of an hour.

It had been weird with Covid so far. Our numbers

had dropped but that almost made it worse for us. We were so used to the department being busy that we were constantly on edge when it was quiet. We had a nagging fear that something bad was going to happen. It usually does.

I've been known to cut patients off when I hear the 'qu' at the start of a word. 'Nooooooo!' I'll yell. 'You can't say that word!' They look at me in astonishment and then I apologize and say we're very superstitious in A&E.

'You're allowed to say it's civilized, or it's looking nice today, or pleasant. You can't say the q word, ever,' I tell them.

This time the forbidden word had slipped out before I had time to stop him. I stitched him up. His hand initially looked like it had been through a meat grinder but it came together quite easily in the end. I spent an hour and a half working on his hand while he slept. I finished at around 6 a.m. just before there was an influx of patients. I was right – that guy had cursed us. I got a rush of adrenalin and knew I had to switch on. I'm always aware that as the night shift goes on, I need to triple check everything I do.

I got home and collapsed into bed knowing that in less than twenty-four hours, I'd have to get up at 5.15 a.m to make it in for a day shift. This schedule was killing me. I had worked sixty hours that week and was ready for a rest. There was just one more shift before I had two days off.

It started with a man who had been drinking fifteen beers a day for the past two weeks.

'Why have you started drinking more?' I asked him.

'Well, because of all this coronavirus stuff that's been going on. I've been drinking to try and relax and pass the time because I'm worried and there isn't much else to do,' he replied.

I guess he must have been one of the individuals I'd heard about on the news earlier who was drinking more during the pandemic than before it had started. He was getting heartburn and reflux symptoms. I gave him some Gaviscon, which you can buy anywhere, and off he went.

At this point in early May, I was seeing more complaints linked to excessive consumption of alcohol. I'd noticed it among friends as well – on video chats they talked about how much more they were drinking. Everyone was doing it. Even I was – I made cocktails with Ed one evening to pass the time, which was a lot of fun. Seriously though, I had started to consciously remind myself when at home that I didn't need to have a drink and that it was better to go without. Even so, I could understand why more people were turning to alcohol.

The shift was broken up by supervision with one of my consultants who was working from home. Our session was done over a video call. I was relieved that I didn't have him standing over me watching me treat patients like he would normally, as that can be quite intimidating. He kept changing the background of the chat and asking me which photo was best. There he was standing on a mountain, then in the Amazon and then on a beach. He chose the beach in the end to lighten the mood.

When my shift ended, I cycled home in anticipation of the next season of *Grey's Anatomy* that had just been released. I could not wait to get started. I love medical dramas, but only the good kind. Those ones which portray CPR in an unrealistic way and promote the thought that it's almost always successful are so unrealistic and can misinform the public. In A&E, we certainly can't shock everyone's hearts back into a working condition. It's important that people realize that.

7

Fed Up with Lockdown

Amid all the coronavirus chaos was VE Day, on 8 May – the seventy-fifth anniversary of the marking of the end of World War II. It was a bank holiday and the country was bathed in glorious sunshine. Street parties that were meant to take place with social distancing measures were happening everywhere with bunting, baking, barbecues and beers. Or that's what I imagined; I was at work. I knew the British public and what they would be up to though, especially after my eight years in A&E. The department is a great place to get an idea of what is going on in society, and I knew people loved an excuse for a good time and a drink or three. As predicted, it wasn't long before the injuries started rolling in in the early after-noon.

One man came in by ambulance. He was aggressive, thrashing around, shouting and trying to get off his trolley. I called security for back up. The paramedics told me that he had been drinking beers all day, fallen over in the garden and hit his head on the patio.

Suddenly, before my eyes, he started to lose consciousness and stopped breathing. I called for an anaesthetist, who rapidly intubated and ventilated him. He was quiet at last, but this was not a good sign. We did a scan of his head and it showed a bleed on the brain. He needed an intensive care bed in the unit that was almost full, caring for Covid patients. He got one but if it weren't for the fact that the hospital had created extra intensive care capacity, the situation would have been very different.

My next four shifts saw an increase in the numbers of patients attending A&E. Did I miss the announcement that lockdown had been lifted? Government advice was still stating that people stay at home.

'So what's brought you into A&E today?' I asked one patient.

'Calf pain,' he replied.

'And how long have you had this calf pain?'

'Seven weeks.'

'Why didn't you come in seven weeks ago?'

'Because of this whole coronavirus thing.'

I busied myself with doing my assessment while withholding the massive sigh that was waiting to escape. A pandemic was still on the loose, after all. Had I woken up in a parallel universe where everything was back to normal? The scenes in hospitals in the US, particularly New York, were frightening and Brazil was also in the grips of the coronavirus crisis. In the UK, around 3,000 new cases were being reported each day.

'The pain came on while I was sat watching television,' he continued. 'It bothers me every now and then.'

His calf looked and felt normal. When I touched it, he felt no pain. There was no history of trauma and I didn't see how an X-ray would help. I spoke to my senior who told me to send him home because there was nothing wrong.

'But what is it?' the patient asked when I went back with the news.

'In all honesty, I'm not sure. But I'm happy there's nothing drastic going on here.'

This wasn't a problem for A&E. I understand patients want answers but we often don't have them. Medicine is a well-informed guessing game sometimes.

I left work and was pleasantly surprised to see Ed standing near my bike. He'd cycled to the hospital to give me some company on the journey home. How sweet, I thought. On the way back, the chain came off his bike. He quickly fixed it, got back on and started pedalling. I was a few metres in front and was just getting my foot clipped in to the pedal when a sudden pain erupted in my buttocks. My husband had crashed into me. He hadn't been looking where he was going.

'Ow!' I yelled. 'That hurt!'

'Oh sorry, I thought you would have got moving by the time I caught up.'

His original good deed was undone and he was in my bad books.

I often try to cycle to and from work because it clears my head. In the morning cycling wakes me up and invigorates me for the day ahead and when I finish work it helps me to decompress. At that time I could only do it on day shifts because twilight shifts saw me finish at midnight and I was too tired. I drove otherwise, but even this wasn't particularly safe after a night shift.

I've woken up before to someone beeping behind me because the traffic lights had turned green and I'd fallen asleep at the wheel. There have been so many times where my head's done a jolt and I momentarily panic. I used to phone Mum and Dad because I knew they'd be up at that time in the morning so that they could keep me talking until I got home. I always wind the windows down and pinch my face. I usually leave without going to the toilet so my bladder is full, in the hope that the discomfort will keep me awake.

It's become easier over the years, but falling asleep at the wheel after a night shift is a real danger for healthcare professionals. When I was a student nurse on intensive care, I found out that two nurses had died within the last couple of months on the way home in the morning after work. As a result everyone was made to eat toast and drink tea before they left. Everyone at work is aware of it. We joke about it, but it's not funny.

I woke up the next morning and my left buttock was really sore. I checked it out in the mirror and saw that it was black and blue. I cursed Ed under my breath for crashing into me on his bike yesterday. Then I grabbed something to eat, left the house and somehow managed, despite some not insignificant discomfort, to cycle into work. On my journey in, my water bottle fell out of its holder onto the road. I stopped and saw it was broken so I went back to pick up the pieces and was annoyed for the rest of the ride in.

I got into work and took a shower. While I was enjoying the water pummelling my back I heard a sudden crashing sound before something sharp hit the back of my ankles. I looked around and three tiles had fallen off the shower wall and lay shattered around my feet. The last thing I needed now, just before my shift, was to step on one, cut my feet and have to be stitched up by a colleague. I hoped nothing else bad was going to happen that day, for the sake of my patients.

My first case was a woman who wasn't answering when my nursing colleagues were calling her name. She had come in after falling and hitting her head on a table corner so it wasn't completely out of the question that she could be unconscious. The only thing was she had already come round and had been awake a little while earlier. As I looked her over I saw her peek at me through a slit in her eyelids to see what was happening. I said her name. There was no response. I tried to move her arm but she resisted. I tried to open her eyelids but she was tensing them shut. She certainly wasn't unconscious, but why was she feigning it? Maybe she just didn't want to be bothered. That was reassuring. I went to check her blood pressure and she suddenly grabbed my arm with one hand, before taking a swing and punching me in the face with the other. Her eyes were half closed and it wasn't a forceful punch, so luckily it didn't hurt and I wasn't left with a bruise. She then dug her nails in and pulled my arm towards her with teeth bared to bite. I quickly did an arm twisting manoeuvre to break her hold, a move I had learnt in training. I was surprised I remembered how to do it under pressure.

'Don't bite me! That's not very nice,' I said.

She went back to pretending to be unconscious again. I couldn't carry out a full assessment so had no choice but to admit her to hospital for further observations. What a wonderful start to the day.

When I joined A&E, I had training on how to get out of a confrontation. I was taught to cross my arms in front of me, take a step back and shout forcefully, 'Get back!' This was meant to stop a man coming at me with a knife. I wasn't sure how effective it would be. Luckily, whenever something like that has looked like it might happen, one of my colleagues has come to my aid and pinned the person up against the wall before they could do anything. It's usually security; they're so great. Later on in my career, I was taught how to get out of a wrist hold and we had some training on how to communicate with an aggressive patient.

Other than that, I've learnt on the job, mainly through making mistakes and experiencing what happened when I said the wrong thing. The last thing you say to someone who is screaming their head off at you is, 'Calm down,' yet it's the first utterance that comes out of your mouth when you're new to it all.

Now I watch people who don't have much experience make the exact same mistakes as I did. The patient gets more and more hot headed and rage ensues. It's quite funny to watch. It might sound cruel, but I need a bit of entertainment now and then and, anyway, sometimes if you go in to help it makes it worse, because from the patient's perspective it looks like a wall of people is coming at them.

The worst example of me making someone angry was probably the man who rang the police telling them that he was going to kill me. I had probably told him to calm down when he was already really angry. Big mistake.

There's no one rule for dealing with angry patients. I try and figure out what it is they're so vexed by. Sometimes it's helpful to say I've been through the same thing and to share stories, but sometimes it's not. If I know a bit about the patient, such as the fact they have children for example, I can try and bring that in to the conversation. Even that has gone horribly wrong for me, though.

Years ago, there was one woman I was treating who was thoroughly unpleasant to me. She was one of our regulars who attended with back pain and had a specific plan of care made by the spinal team with regular follow-up dates in the diary. She wasn't taking her medications, was a regular cannabis user and a difficult case for us to manage as an emergency department – there was little more we could do to help her. On this occasion, she was there with some of her kids. She laid on the A&E trolley busily tapping away on her phone while her four children were running around causing chaos. As her pain seemed well controlled and the doctor was happy for her to be discharged, it was my responsibility to aid her out of the department, but she refused to leave. Every second word was a profanity or an insult, and it got to the point where I couldn't take much more.

'This isn't setting a good example for your children,' I said.

She went apoplectic with rage. A torrent of swear words came out of her mouth and her face turned a deep shade of red.

'This behaviour and attitude you have is impacting on their lives,' I added. Her children should have been at school.

'You've got some of your children here. Why are they here?' I continued. 'They shouldn't be witnessing this argument that is completely unnecessary between you and me. Let's have a calm, grown-up conversation.'

Looking back, this was obviously completely the wrong way to have handled this situation, as her reaction told me.

'You don't know anything! You don't have any fucking children,' she said, before she spewed out another stream of vile language and insults.

Making judgemental comments about her as a mother was the wrong thing to do. I maintain though that her behaviour was disgusting. Her oldest child had started to imitate her and was swearing at me too, which was a worrying sign.

Occasionally, no matter what I do, there's a fundamental personality clash with a patient. It rarely happens, but sometimes it's best to leave, let their fury subside, before sending a colleague in who can level with them. These confrontations leave *me* angry too, but then I think that I can't get through to everybody. There will always be people who will have different opinions and life values.

It can be frustrating, because as health workers, part of our mission is to give everyone the best care and advice regarding how to improve their health. I see people taking bad decisions that will impact on their health, but I remind myself that it's their right to do so and that I can't help everybody. It doesn't mean I don't stop trying, though.

My cycle into work the next day was bracing because it was so chilly. The temperature had suddenly dropped ten degrees overnight. I was in isolation and thankful for once for the extra layer of protection and warmth. The first patient of the day was pregnant. Pregnant women make me nervous because there are two lives to take care of instead of just one. She was really short of breath and complaining of chest pain. Although her symptoms were linked to Covid, I wasn't sure she had the virus. Pregnant women are at risk of blood clots that can sit in the vessels around the lungs. It's called a pulmonary embolism, or PE for short. I'd seen a few cases of pregnant women with PEs from over the years and they were high-octane medical situations that were frightening for everyone involved.

One woman who was heavily pregnant had PEs on both her lungs and was really close to arresting. She was struggling to breathe and looked terrified. I was working with a colleague to give her a drug that would break up the clots. You have to get the dosage exactly right because too much can cause a person to bleed out, so naturally I was taking my time to make sure I got everything correct. The registrar in charge is one of my favourite people to work with. He's so calm and collected, and nothing fazes him. Around him there can be total chaos, but he maintains a clear head and knows exactly what to do. Attending a cardiac arrest with him is like sitting down for a cup of tea. On that occasion though, even he snapped at me to hurry up because he was stressed and nervous too. Luckily, we got the dosage right, and she and baby came out the other side.

This time, however, I was the one in charge of spotting whether the woman had a PE and making the decisions. Questions were running through my head. If the woman arrested, what would happen? Would the baby survive? Would I have to phone Obstetrics to get them to do an emergency C-section and deliver the baby while a team of us tried to resuscitate the mother? That scenario had played out in A&E before; the baby survived but the mother didn't. I was suddenly feeling very hot inside my PPE.

What made the situation worse was that the scanner we would normally use was temporarily out of action. Either she waited a couple of days, or she could get a CT scan, which involved a lot more radiation and meant the patient was at increased risk of breast cancer. I explained the risks and the benefits and asked her what she would like to do.

'What would you do?' she asked.

I dread that question. It really wasn't my place to say. Even if I did opine, my decision wouldn't necessarily be the right one for her. I wasn't pregnant, I'd never had children so couldn't put myself in her shoes. For that reason, I never give opinions because I don't know everything about someone's life, it's not appropriate. But it's always an awful situation when this happens because the patient wants guidance; they see the health-care professional before them as someone who has more knowledge, experience of these matters and clinical expertise. In cases like these I almost feel obstructive. I saw the turmoil she was in, so repeated the pros and cons of each decision and hoped I had been helpful in some way. She opted to wait and so I admitted her to be observed overnight.

I followed her up and her scan had revealed that it was indeed a PE which had subsequently been treated.

All was well. Phew. Her case represented a wider problem that we were starting to come up against, however. She had been admitted to an isolation unit for Covid patients. Luckily, because numbers had started to drop, we had one that was free and it had just been deep cleaned. It had been just me and her alone in there, which was highly unusual. What if she had come in a few weeks earlier when all our isolation units were being used and were near full? The situation could have been very different. Would she have caught Covid on top of everything else? Probably not, though I can't guarantee it.

As a team, we were having to make really tough decisions as to where to treat patients. So many symptoms could potentially have been Covid, but then they might not have been. We were still seeing all the normal health problems that were going on before coronavirus came into our lives. Should we admit them to the hot area or the cold one? If the patient didn't have Covid but was admitted to a hot area because the person triaging them thought their symptoms matched up with the virus, their chances of contracting it were higher. If you admitted them to a cold area and they ended up having Covid, that presented a risk to other patients and staff, lots of whom were working there because they themselves were either pregnant or had underlying health conditions that meant they were more vulnerable. It was a constant see-saw of a debate and it was mentally strenuous and difficult to always have to be thinking of this new aspect of patient care, on top of everything else.

While on my way to the next patient, one of the senior members of nursing staff came up to me to inspect the goggles I had on as part of my PPE. The trust had been notified of deliveries of substandard equipment that needed to be recalled. It reminded me of times in the past when mobile phone companies have had to recall products that have spontaneously combusted. Except this was meant to prevent me from contracting a virus that could kill me and others. I had to laugh. It was that or be sucked down a whirlpool of despair.

My trust had acted really quickly in getting the message out there, but who knew how long this faulty equipment had been in circulation before they were informed? They bombarded us with emails, put screensavers on all the computers, used pop up messages to make sure everyone was aware. People were deployed around the trust to check every single member of staff working and tell them to get out of the isolation area if they weren't kitted out with the correct PPE.

I went home and had a video chat with my mum and sister who were still in lockdown together. The last time I had seen them in the flesh was at my father's service of thanksgiving three months earlier. I knew Mum was still grieving. My sister told me she had been making her infamous Mars Bar cake and giving it to the neighbours.

I felt upset that I couldn't see my mum and sister, and a pang of jealousy when I saw friends on social media meeting up with their relatives, albeit at a two-metre distance, as government guidance was stating at the time.

On 10 May, Prime Minister Boris Johnson made his announcement on the next stage of lockdown. It left the country more confused than ever. Was I now allowed to see my mum and sister? I didn't know. In any case, I was still worried about passing on coronavirus. I was a risky person to be around but I also knew that if I'd had it, then I would have passed symptoms on to Ed and neither of us had experienced anything but full health so far. If anything, I thought I might have had coronavirus back in December before we really knew much about it. I'd felt off colour for a few days, which was rare for me. Either way, I'd never know.

I also thought I was safe at work; it's very common practice for me to have good hand hygiene. Other people didn't understand how germs spread; for example from touching their supermarket trolley, then their phone and finally their face. Also, if I did decide to see people, I definitely wasn't going to break the rules, because I really didn't want to hurt anybody.

The next day at work, I saw another person with chest pain. He was in his early thirties; his observations were all OK. I wanted to rule out the possibility of a PE, as he was describing a pain that sounded more like it was coming from the lungs rather than the heart. His blood test looked like I might be right and he went for a scan, which confirmed it. I couldn't believe it. He had no risk factors such as being pregnant, he wasn't a smoker and he hadn't had a recent hospital admission, which are usually the main causes. That was two patients in close succession that had had PEs. I gave him some drugs and he was admitted to hospital. These were among the first PEs I had treated since starting in my new role as an ACP.

My next patient had been passing stools that looked like black tar. He had had gastric ulcers in the past and looked pale.

'Are you normally this pale?' I asked, hoping he wouldn't take offence.

'I don't think so,' he replied.

His heart was racing. I phoned the gastroenterology department as I was pretty sure that he had a bleed somewhere in his gut. I went back and told him, 'We're going to have to admit you.'

'Oh no, no, no. I'm not coming in. I don't want to catch the virus,' he said quickly.

'I sympathize with your concerns but if you go home, you will most likely continue to bleed and become more unwell. You're already at a critical point, your heart is beating faster.'

I didn't say much more because I knew it was his life and his decision, so I left to give him a bit of time to think.

There are often times when patients don't do what we advise. Some people are mostly fine but we just want to check a few things and would like them to stay a bit longer. Sometimes they'll say they'd rather just go home, which is not a big problem. Those patients who take overdoses and want to go home are a bit more complex. We have to judge whether they have capacity to decide. If we let them go, will they kill themselves? Are they still under the influence of whatever they've taken? Sometimes we judge that they shouldn't be making this decision in the state they're in and then have to physically restrain them from leaving. That is really difficult and a very controversial area of healthcare. We try to judge each situation as best we can and always have the interests of the patient at the forefront of everything. I understand that this kind of situation can be hugely traumatic for the patient though – that's why it's so hard.

At the other end of the spectrum, there are the patients who know they're going to die, from terminal cancer for example. Medical professionals naturally want to do as much as they can to prolong life but sometimes the person on the receiving end has had enough. People in a sound state of mind are allowed to do what they want and we let them, however hard and upsetting it is for us to stand back and not do anything. I always say to myself: 'I'm letting this person go and they're going to die but they have terminal cancer, so that is going to happen anyway. Why should I prolong their suffering when they don't want to continue living with it?' I think about what the kindest thing to do is, and am always guided by senior clinicians.

I went back to see my patient. 'I've reconsidered and agree to come in,' he told me. Thank God for that.

As I moved away I realized that A&E had suddenly become busy. All the cubicles were full and patients were starting to gather in the middle of the majors section of the department. The situation was so bad that management had appeared. Hospital managers are a bit mysterious; no one seems to know exactly who they are and sometimes they don't introduce themselves by name, but instead a code title, like gold, silver or bronze. They are on our side, but there's very occasionally a bit of tension between managers and clinicians where there is a clash of opinions.

Once someone in a suit appeared in front of me and started wheeling my patient out of resus.

'Excuse me, who are you and what are you doing with my patient?' I asked, slightly alarmed that someone seemed to be kidnapping the person I was meant to be looking after.

'They're about to breach. I'm taking them up to the ward,' they replied.

'Hmm, OK, but they've got a low blood pressure so they need to stay here.'

He paused for a second and then sighed in frustration before he turned the patient back around and walked off.

I knew this breach, where a patient had been in A&E

longer than targets dictated, would cost the hospital a lot of money, but patient safety always comes first.

I completely understand that a manager's job is to help both clinicians and patients. Management had done so well with the crisis and a whole incident team had been put together to oversee the hospital's response to coronavirus. We hadn't been overwhelmed. When we are drowning as a department, with too many patients, they are always there helping. Like me, their priority is patient care but there is a slight difference in how they look at things.

I'm also aware that they take a lot of heat from higher up. It starts at a national level when A&Es are struggling in winter and not meeting targets, for example, and then runs right down to the clinicians. By the time the anger and annoyance gets to us, it's been diluted to such an extent that we barely feel it. We are shielded from a lot of what goes on higher up the food chain. The managers are incredible people and I don't envy their jobs.

On this occasion, their appearance in A&E was because they were worried that social distancing measures were not in place, so they asked us to make plans for our patients to be moved on as quickly as possible. Management were chasing beds on the wards so they could be taken out of A&E. It was really important to keep hospital flow moving and to avoid A&E getting too clogged up. We were still a risky area, despite every possible precaution that had been taken.

*   *   *

During the weeks when anxiety around coronavirus was at its peak and patient numbers had dwindled, leaving A&E a pleasant and calm place to work, management had been working on improvement projects. They were determined that the department was not going to revert to the way it was during the winter pressures, with patients stuck in A&E unable to move because there were no beds available. I was always sceptical and now it looked like I would be proved right. Already we had started to see a small but steady stream of patients trickling back in with problems that they should have been seeing their GP about. I didn't see how they were going to stop the trickle turning into a flood and all the usual problems returning. I didn't know how they planned to prevent long waiting times and patients being stuck in A&E, but there was some suggestion of empowering staff to be able to turn patients away and tell them to visit an urgent care centre or their GP instead. Those places would be more equipped and, in theory, have more time to deal with minor health problems than us.

8

She's Alive!

I had come in early, as usual, to check the status of every patient I had seen. Those seconds while I sat and watched the computer whir into life were a vacuum in time, hope and dread suspended for a brief moment before the reality of their outcome hit me and I was brought back to earth with a bump. My thoughts turned to Shirley, the woman with Covid-19 who had deteriorated in fifteen minutes and who I had sent to intensive care, wishing her luck and not knowing what the future held. As far as I knew, she was still on the unit. Would today be the day I found out she had become another victim to the virus? I waited with bated breath as her hospital records loaded. I saw a discharge letter. I couldn't believe it. She had survived Covid-19 and was alive! I was so relieved, and happy. What a great start to the day this was. It was a miracle that she had not become one of the figures on the trust's daily emails stating how many people had been admitted as well as those who had died.

I wanted to celebrate, but of course it wasn't

appropriate, so did a mini jig in my chair. I then thought that we should mark the positives in this crisis more. All anyone seemed to hear about was death. I'd seen one video of someone being clapped off the ward, but I craved more.

At the same time, however, I was more than aware of how coronavirus was sweeping the UK's care homes. I work with them quite a bit in my job and saw variations in how they set themselves up to protect residents and staff from becoming ill. My godmother had been stuck in her room for weeks after testing positive for the virus. She was fed up with not being able to see anyone, but had not deteriorated with any of the symptoms. This was a miracle in itself. Mum told me she had finally been allowed to sit in the garden after testing negative. There had been stories of care workers who had left their families and moved in with residents to shield everyone. Others had isolated all their residents in their rooms and this had its consequences.

One elderly man had come into A&E feeling suicidal after staying in his room for weeks. He had been separated from his wife next door and the impact on his mental health had been detrimental. I was scared more generally that the older generations were being forgotten and I worried that people didn't seem to care. A patient told me: 'Ah well, you know this coronavirus is only going to affect one part of the population from now on. The rest of us should just carry on as normal.' I seethed with inner rage. It felt like he was saying that we should let coronavirus wipe a segment of the population out.

Every life matters, and I was dismayed that not everyone seemed to see that.

That day I was in the isolation unit. It was full but it was the only one open out of three. This was great news and reassuring. It looked like we were over the worst of it. I hoped care homes were also seeing a decline in people with coronavirus.

There wasn't much time to stop and think as the paramedics came in with a patient. He had a very high temperature but that's all anyone knew about him. It was hard to find out more as he was confused, combative and telling me to 'fuck off' as he lashed out. Before I knew it, he had landed a punch on my shoulder; I hadn't managed to move out the way quick enough.

A good history is key in establishing what is going on with someone. In this case, without one, I could only consider what his temperature might mean. It could be a sign of infection, possibly Covid. I ordered a chest X-ray, which looked clear, but that didn't necessarily rule Covid out. The results from his blood test pointed towards it being an infection, but I didn't know what the source of it was. One thing was for sure, he needed to come in, so I referred him to a consultant. Neither of us was sure whether it was coronavirus or not and we wouldn't get the swab result for another twenty-four hours. This was another example of the constant debate we were faced with. Wherever we put him, someone was at risk, whether it was the patient or other staff.

Another patient was brought in who was complaining of shortness of breath. His stomach was swollen and he was the colour of Homer Simpson. He had a type of liver disease and his tummy had been increasing in size over the past couple of weeks. It was likely to be an abnormal build-up of fluid in the abdomen. I wasn't surprised he was feeling short of breath; the pressure of the fluid must have been so uncomfortable. He had no other Covid symptoms so I quickly admitted him to a cold area of the hospital to get the fluid drained.

On to my next patient, and she was describing classic coronavirus symptoms. For the past week she had been feeling tired with aching muscles, and feverish with a persistent cough. She was a walking advert for the virus, but looked too well for us to be worried about her. She had walked in to see us that day. Her oxygen levels were excellent and the rest of her observations were stable too. She definitely didn't need to be admitted.

'You're fine to go home and ride this out,' I said. 'No point in you staying in hospital.'

'But what if it's the virus? You can't just expect me to go home!' she shouted, at such a volume that everybody could hear every word.

The surrounding hustle and bustle suddenly stopped and was replaced by silence as my colleagues waited to hear how I would de-escalate the rapidly building tension.

'Your oxygen levels are great. You don't need any extra. You can certainly manage these symptoms at home; we really can't do anything more for you. It's definitely a good thing that you don't need to come in.'

'But I think I should come in. I feel like you're sending me home to my death!'

'I've done every test necessary and you are in good health apart from these symptoms you're displaying. Home is the best place for you right now.'

I somehow wasn't managing to get through to this patient. 'What can I do to make you feel better?' I asked her.

'You need to bring me into hospital,' she answered.

'I've already explained that can't happen so how else can I reassure you?'

'Bring me into hospital!'

'We're going round in circles now. You can't come in and that's final.'

She left, but she was not happy about it and mumbled and muttered on her way out. I checked in with my conscience. Had I done the right thing? I turned towards my consultant who had heard the whole showdown. 'That was the right thing to do,' he told me before I had opened my mouth to ask.

I cycled home, exhausted from the confrontations I'd had at work that day. They always took a lot out of me because I had to be on high alert and work out how to manage the situation as best I could. Ed and I settled down to watch a new series that had just come out, but it wasn't long before I passed out on the sofa with the lights on at 8.30 p.m.

The next day I woke up to news saying there had been an increase in coronavirus cases in my local area since the latest phase of releasing lockdown had happened on 10 May. Below the article were comments along the lines of, 'I told you so.' I wasn't sure I had seen this reflected in the number of inpatient cases in our daily bulletins from the trust. In any case, it didn't make sense for there to have been a sudden increase so soon after the prime minister's speech. It didn't stop the niggling worry I felt, though, as I set off on my bike ride to work.

When I got in, I was assigned to minors and saw a patient who hadn't opened his bowels, or even passed wind, in ten days. It's incredibly important to do a poo. It can be dangerous if you don't and can cause a great deal of discomfort and, in the worst case, death.

I sent him for a scan which ruled out anything sinister like a perforated bowel, which would see bits of faecal matter escape and cause infection. He was just severely constipated. I did a rectal examination and gave him an enema – an injection of fluid into the lower bowel – at the same time. I hoped that would get things moving.

'Here's a commode for you, let's hope you manage to go to the toilet. I'll come back and check on you,' I said.

I kept going back at regular intervals. 'Anything yet?'
'No, no,' he replied.

'Hmmmm, hopefully it won't be too long now,' I said.

It was a good hour before anything happened and when it did it was a massive relief. His tummy was so swollen and he was in a lot of pain. To have that release of opening his bowels after ten days must have been the best feeling ever, and so satisfying.

'Well done!' I said. I meant it, I was so proud. In A&E we take all the small things as an achievement. I had made a big difference to this man's life and I felt great. After that poo, he went home with more laxatives to keep things moving.

Next up was a woman who said she was dizzy. I hate this word and am always on edge whenever someone mentions it. It can mean so many things, from the benign to the fatal. I asked her what she meant by 'dizzy'. She looked at me like I was stupid and like I should know because I was the medical professional in the room.

'Something is not right, I just know it.'

Now I was really on edge. This was one of those phrases that ring alarm bells in my head.

'How long have you been dizzy for?' I asked.

'Four days. And I've had a headache too,' she replied. 'My boyfriend says I've been acting weirdly.'

Her boyfriend had dropped her off and was sat outside in the car park waiting, so I called him to find out more. Visitors still weren't allowed in the hospital except in really special circumstances, like if someone was dying.

'She's been behaving oddly for the past few days,' he said. 'Things like calling everyday objects the wrong name, and forgetting where the cutlery goes.'

It was enough to convince me to perform a scan of her head which showed she had a bleed around the brain. That indicated that it was time for the neuro-surgeons to take over.

The rest of the day was taken up with four patients, all complaining of chest pain. They all started blurring into one. One patient's pain extended into their right arm, another's went into their left. One patient described the pain as sharp while the other said it was like an elephant was sitting on their chest. None of the tests I did showed anything to worry about so I concluded these were more people with coronavirus anxiety.

The following shift was also defined by chest pain, albeit one that turned out to have more immediately life-threatening connotations. I walked in to see a fifty-year-old woman who had been experiencing pain on and off for a week but had decided to ignore it. To me, it was so obviously cardiac chest pain, possibly a heart attack, but she thought it was indigestion.

Although many people who turn up in A&E want to know they haven't had a heart attack, there are just as many who experience one and leave it too late to come in. Heart attacks can be easy to miss. They are a build-up of plaque in the blood vessels around the heart which eventually leads to a blockage. If blood cannot get through to the other side there's no oxygen going through either, and so the tissue dies. To solve the problem, stents – small balloons that open up vessels – are inserted. People can have a mild heart attack, but if it's one of the big vessels that is blocked, they may well die.

Whenever I hear someone complain of chest pain, I explain that it could be one of a number of problems. From an A&E point of view, the most concerning things to look out for are a heart attack, clots, pneumonia or a dissecting aorta.

'I don't think your aorta has dissected,' I told her. 'There's no infection because your chest sounds clear. I don't think it's a clot on your lungs. That leaves a potential heart attack. We will do some blood tests to find out. Do you have any other concerns or questions I can help you with?'

'How long have I got?' she came back with.

I paused. She said it in such a serious tone that I thought I had a patient who was really worried on my hands. She suddenly started laughing. I tried to join in with her, but it was very half hearted. I didn't really think we should be laughing about what would turn out to be a very real heart attack.

In complete contrast to that patient with her jovial attitude was the person I saw in the isolation unit the next day. He had had a CT scan which showed signs of Covid-19. I went to tell him the results and his response caught me completely off guard.

'So, I'm going to die,' he said.

'What makes you think that?' I asked.

I didn't think he was anywhere near being a serious case of coronavirus but I had learnt to never give patients definite answers when there aren't any. It's the same with promises. I never promise anything because nine times out of ten, I won't be able to fulfil it. You never know what's round the corner in A&E and patients can deteriorate rapidly out of the blue and when nobody was expecting it.

'Well, I have diabetes and asthma, and I'm over sixty,' he replied. 'So that means I'm going to die.'

He was being deadly serious. I put my hand on his arm as he started to cry.

'There have been hundreds of patients in this hospital alone who have been discharged back to their homes after testing positive for the virus and being admitted to one of the wards,' I said. 'Your oxygen levels are good and you look well. I'm even happy for you to go home.'

His fear took me aback, but I'd seen it so many times in people with suspected or confirmed Covid. Where had it come from? What kind of messages were the general public receiving?

My next patient was elderly and had been found by their care worker in the morning, collapsed on the lounge floor. He had been there for hours and excrement was surrounding him. The care worker had told the paramedics that he seemed more confused than normal.

'Do you remember what happened to you?' I asked.

'No, nothing. Why am I here?'

He had a diagnosis of dementia and obviously didn't know what had occurred. We had been warned that many older patients who were later diagnosed with Covid-19 were presenting with diarrhoea and confusion, instead of the more traditional cough, shortness of breath and fever. I didn't think he was well enough to go home so admitted him onto a ward where our specialist older people's health team would take care of him.

Moments later, I pulled back the curtain and saw my next patient – a skeleton of a man laid out on the bed in front of me.

'Hello, my name's Louise. What's brought you in to A&E today?'

'I've been short of breath for a couple of months but it's really got worse in the last couple of weeks. I used to be able to walk for miles, but now I can hardly manage the length of my garden,' he said.

I looked at his chart and saw that his GP had given him antibiotics for a chest infection that my patient said hadn't helped his health at all.

'I've also lost a lot of weight over the past few months,' he added.

Although he had symptoms that suggested Covid-19, I had a horrible feeling that something much more sinister was at play. The CT scan confirmed that my instincts were right. His body was riddled with cancer. I was gutted. He was the main carer for his wife, who had dementia. I arranged for extra care to be provided for her because he needed to be brought into hospital.

I went back to tell him and he asked, 'Why are you bringing me in?'

'Your scan has shown some abnormalities. It could be cancer but I need to admit you so my colleagues can carry out further investigations and explore with you what's really wrong,' I answered.

I knew it was definitely cancer but I couldn't say that to the patient. The process of breaking bad news had to be handled so delicately and I didn't think it right to tell him what I had found out. I wasn't the best person to answer any follow-up questions he would almost certainly have. In my mind, it would be doing him a disservice, a bit like dropping a china tea cup, seeing it shatter when it hit the ground, and then having to rush off before I could pick up the pieces. That wouldn't be fair and it was better for a specialist who knew much more about the intricacies of his cancer to sit down with him and explore his options. I was delaying the truth for just a short while.

By this time I had been in PPE for seven hours straight having drunk nothing and not gone to the toilet. It was my own fault. I had kept saying to myself, 'Oh, I'll just quickly see one more patient.' Before I knew it, all that time had gone by. I was walking past when one of the patients stopped me in my tracks. 'Are you hungry? Your stomach is making loud rumbles,' they said. Time to eat. I handed over the patients I was looking after to the fresh-faced doctors who had just started their shifts before I escaped for some much needed fresh air and food.

Just as I was walking out of the unit, a patient was rushed in vomiting blood. It looked like something out of a horror film. She was covered in blood and the bowl she was vomiting into was already overflowing and spilling everywhere. I hesitated. Did they need extra help? No, a group of my colleagues had run towards her and were on track to do everything they could for her.

I couldn't wait to take my mask off outside. I can only describe the feeling as the one you might get when taking off a T-shirt drenched with sweat after a hot, busy and stressful day before jumping into a pool. Except this was better. The mask peeled off my face leaving an indentation across my cheeks where it had sucked at my skin for however long it had been on. Finally I felt fresh air skim over my face, which had had sweat pouring over and down it non-stop for hours. It was absolute bliss.

9

Alcohol Is Terrifying

After much confusion, I had got to the bottom of the new government guidelines and had worked out that I was allowed to meet one person at a time outside while keeping a distance of two metres between us. It didn't take me long to call a friend I hadn't seen for a month since she parked up outside my house and stood on the pavement holding up some balloons and a sign saying happy birthday. She joined me on my dog walk and after getting over the initial awkwardness of not being able to hug, we spent the next couple of hours strolling through fields in the sunshine. We discussed how we were both coping in lockdown; she had been doing lots of yoga, reading books and cooking. She'd also given her boyfriend a questionable haircut. I told her that my husband had got so sick of his shaggy hair that he had shaved it all off himself.

As we walked, I had to stop whenever my dog Max did a poo and look at it closely. His stools had remnants of a Tesco bag for life in them that he had munched on over the weekend. I was worried that he had eaten it in desperation because he had worms, which would make him hungrier than normal.

I tend to treat my dogs as if they are my patients sometimes. A few years ago, when we had just got our first dog, we went for a walk and she came charging back to us after running off after a squirrel. She didn't see the barbed-wire fence in the way, ran straight through it and sliced her ear in two. We were an hour away from home and her ear dripped with blood the whole way back. She kept shaking her head because her ear was bothering her and I soon had her blood splattered all over my face, hair and clothes. Back at the house, I found an expired supply of medical glue and stuck her flapping ear back together. The scar is still visible now but I was pretty pleased with how it healed.

I said goodbye to my friend and returned home with the dogs. It was twenty-seven degrees outside and the hottest day of the year so far. I really hoped that I wouldn't be in the isolation unit that day, where I would have to wear PPE and no doubt sweat even more profusely than I usually did in it.

Thankfully I was in majors. I can't tell you how relieved I was when the consultant told me in the roll call. I felt sorry for my colleagues who would be working in isolation, but I knew they'd only be sent in there for short periods.

My first patient was brought in after a passer-by had found her collapsed on the street. She had an extensive history of drug abuse and was drifting in and out of consciousness. All I could get from her was that her head hurt. She might have been under the influence of heroin; I saw multiple injection marks on her arms and legs but I needed to make sure this was just the effect of drugs and nothing else. Could she have meningitis or encephalitis, or even a bleed on the brain? I scanned her head and it showed a significant bleed. She needed theatre urgently.

The next task was to get a cannula in so that we could give her medicine. Her veins were so shot from having injected drugs into them over such a long period of time that trying to find a good one proved very difficult. Eventually I discovered a vein hidden on the inside of her arm. Not the traditional place to put a cannula, but no one cared about that. Once that was done, off she went for emergency surgery.

After that dramatic episode, I spent a good half hour phoning a list of numbers on my next patient's phone trying to find out more about why he was in A&E. He was in his fifties but chronic alcohol abuse over a number of years meant he looked decades older. He also looked malnourished and smelt of alcohol and stale urine. He was covered in bruises and groaned when I pressed down on his spine while doing my assessment. Scans of his head and neck came back with no injury but I discovered he had five spinal fractures.

I finally got hold of his mother and introduced myself over the phone. 'He's fallen over several times at home,' she went on to tell me. I presumed this had been when he was stumbling around drunk.

'He's also got evidence of self-harm on his arms. Do you know anything about why he might be doing that?' I asked.

'Yes I do. There's a gang of women who live close by who have been stealing from him. He's vulnerable so they pick on him. One of them is meant to be his girlfriend.'

This girlfriend was clearly financially abusing him. His injuries were bad enough for him to be admitted to hospital. I was glad. At least he'd get a few days of peace and we could talk to him about what was going on and hopefully point him in the direction of some help.

Many people judge those who turn up drunk in the emergency department and call them time wasters. I don't think that's the case and feel deep sympathy for them. They are often plagued by mental health problems and are stuck in a vicious cycle of drinking to make their emotional pain go away. I can guarantee that every one of these 'time wasters' has a history you would not wish on your worst enemy.

Many alcoholics and drug addicts used to live successful lives until something awful happened. Some are former soldiers suffering from post-traumatic stress disorder after seeing terrible things in the army. Others were abused as children. Alcohol and drugs become an escape from the thoughts and memories whirring around on a constant loop in their heads. They numb the pain, even if it's only for a short while.

It's not only alcoholics who come into A&E drunk. First in on a night shift are the students, who turn up before 10 p.m. because they're young, fresh out of school, usually away from home and have gone too hard, too soon. Then you get those who work 9–5 jobs and who tend to go out on a Friday or Saturday. Often, the number of those people is higher on pay day or a bank holiday. On top of that are people who are very well-to-do with a lot of money. They come in wearing a smart suit and have often been at some black tie event. I can tell they're fairly wealthy because their postcodes indicate they live in a very respectable part of town. All of the above usually come in because they've fallen over and hit their head.

Alcohol is terrifying. I've seen a man in his twenties become paralysed after he climbed on someone's shoulders on a night out. His friend stumbled and he fell off and landed on his neck. As he lay in front of me, he kept asking, 'Why can't I feel my legs?' None of us really knew what to say. It was devastating and scary to watch. One moment a couple of hours earlier he had been having fun. The next his life had changed irrevocably.

After seeing things like that, I'm now a bit of a party pooper. I get really annoyed when my friends get too drunk and don't know their limits. I worry when Ed goes out because he's so vulnerable when he gets drunk and I know there are people out there who will take advantage of that. I've heard too many stories of idiots who just go up to someone randomly and punch them across the face. I've seen people die from being punched once. I've also seen people die from 'having a bit of fun' and doing parkour when they've had a few drinks. So many individuals have come in with head injuries from doing something stupid when they were intoxicated and have ended up in intensive care on the border between life and death. That extra shot of tequila or sambuca that often seems a great idea at the time, is often not. It might just make you feel that bit worse in the morning, or it might change your life in ways you could never have predicted when you put the glass to your lips and drank its contents.

We were approaching the end of May and it was definitely starting to feel like we were past the worst of the coronavirus peak in the UK. It wasn't over though, and the World Health Organization had recently issued a stark warning saying the virus was still rife throughout the world. In England, more people were getting tested and so numbers of confirmed cases were still high, but the amount of deaths each day was declining slowly. I was down to work a night shift. I always try and take a nap for a couple of hours in the evening before I go in to the hospital later on. My good intentions don't always go to plan. I had recently been woken by one of the dogs lying on top of my stomach in 24°C heat. This time, it was the clapping and banging of saucepans that stirred me from my slumber in the weekly Clap for our Carers that happened on Thursdays at 8 p.m.

When Covid-19 began turning the world upside down, people in different countries had gathered at a certain time each week to show their collective gratitude to the thousands of people working to keep things moving. The UK also had its version which was set up by a mum in London who wanted to show her appreciation for all the key workers doing their bit. The first Clap for our Carers applause happened on 26 March and it gathered momentum each week afterwards, fast becoming an established part of everybody's lives during lockdown.

I loved it. I found it emotional, so much so that I welled up the first couple of times it happened. I had always been at home for it but saw loads of videos of what happened at work. Rows of ambulances and police cars would line the street outside the hospital with their lights flashing. I found it supportive and it felt like we were finally getting some recognition and thanks. I felt appreciated for the first time. When I went to join in outside my front door, all the neighbours were out and one aimed a clap directly at me because I had treated her mother in A&E before. It had started to get a bit repetitive but I still enjoyed it, and it was a reminder that something was still going on and that everybody was in it together. I had felt, in the past couple of weeks, that people had forgotten we were still in the middle of a pandemic.

That week was slightly marred by a message that had gone out from the trust warning staff that the media were offering a financial reward for a photo of healthcare workers breaking social-distancing rules. I had no idea if it was true, but it had caused unrest among some of those working in the hospital and warning messages were flooding my social media feeds and work email.

I made my way into the hospital and was down to spend the shift in the isolation unit. There was only one open, however, so I was sent to work in minors, where a flurry of patients had all arrived at the same time. It had been another sweltering day so I was glad not to be wearing extensive PPE.

An elderly man had come in with a problem with his catheter. It was blocked and so urine was not draining. He was feeling uncomfortable as his bladder was filling with urine. I quickly found out that a blood clot in his bladder had lodged itself in the way and had caused the obstruction. I sorted it out and felt satisfied that I had attended to this man's problem. While I was fixing his medical issue, he chatted away to me.

'My wife suffered a stroke some years ago and lost her ability to talk as a consequence,' he told me. 'Then she was diagnosed with dementia and is now living in a nursing home. Up until lockdown began, I was going back and forth to see her but I can't do that at the moment.'

I got the sense that he was lonely and wanted someone to talk to. Minors had emptied and there were plenty of staff in, so I made my patient a cup of tea and sat down next to his bed while he regaled me with some of his life stories.

It's so rare to be able to do this in A&E, but as a nurse, I feel that is a huge part of what I should be doing in my job. Nurses are advocates for our patients; we are there for them and the thing we really strive for is to provide the best care we can. That care can be medical and emotional, whether it be giving someone painkillers or antibiotics, or lending an ear for them to offload. This pandemic had, up to a certain point, allowed us to spend more time with patients because so many people had stopped attending A&E. I was happy to be able to help by giving that extra support and being someone who would listen to him. That was important at the time; I'd noticed how many more people were suffering with loneliness during a period where face-to-face interactions were sparse.

My next patient was a woman who had Parkinson's disease.

'I've been falling more,' she told me. 'Three times in the last twenty-four hours and I couldn't get up myself after the last one.'

I got to work assessing her. It could just be a progression of her Parkinson's but she had also spiked a temperature. It wasn't a typical Covid-19 presentation and perhaps that was why she had been admitted into the cold area, but I arranged for her to be transferred to the isolation unit for further investigations into the cause of her many falls.

The rest of my patients that night could have got away with booking an appointment with their GP. There was the woman in her thirties who most likely had a sexually transmitted infection. I couldn't do anything about it so told her to go to a GUM clinic. She was terribly embarrassed, so much so that she was shaking, but she didn't need to be. It's such a common problem. Another patient had scabies. I told them to see the pharmacist to get a cream to treat it.

When I woke up the next morning, I read the daily staff briefing we get by email. Over the last three or four days there hadn't been an increase in the number of deaths from Covid-19 in our hospital. That day the number had gone up. More lives had been lost. I lay in my bed and wondered who they were. Was it someone I had seen and cared for? They had almost certainly passed through A&E. What family had they left behind? They would surely be going through the earth-shattering grief that I had experienced when my dad passed away only a few months before. We never used to hear about how many people died in the hospital before corona-virus hit; my experience would be either their life force left them before my eyes or I would follow up a patient and find out they had gone. It was strange now to sit and think about those individuals. I also felt a bit deflated. With a preceding few days of no increase in deaths, I had thought that Covid-19 might be on its way out. But this rise had brought me back to reality with a bump. I didn't think there would be an end to the pandemic. Instead it would become something we learnt to live with. A vaccine might be developed and then it would be like another flu that people got, that would continue to kill vulnerable people.

I was aware that we were still seriously having to adapt in A&E. For so many years the department had been overcrowded but that would no longer be possible for fear of the virus spreading. If we hit over forty patients in majors, we would have to stop ambulance crews from unloading any more and only admit them on a one out, one in basis. This had already happened at a local hospital which, during winter pressures, was notorious for keeping patients waiting on ambulances for hours. This was why management had started to appear when the department looked like it was getting busy. As long as Covid-19 remained an issue, the way the hospital worked would have to be very different.

Our caution was at odds with how the general public were feeling. It seemed like so many people were seeing a light at the end of the tunnel. There were dates in the diary; the shops were due to open in mid-June. At first you could meet up with one person, then on 1 June it became six. Children were going back to school. For some, life was regaining a bit of normality. In A&E we were in a constant cycle of change; I didn't think we would ever go back to how it was before.

Would people appreciate that and learn to treat A&E as the place only for urgent treatment and emergencies like it was meant to be? At my most cynical, I doubted it. During winter pressures, news bulletins were filled with stories about how overcrowded and under pressure emergency departments across the country were, but that didn't stop the tides of patients who could have sought treatment elsewhere from coming in. Some people would even joke when they came in with a complaint they should have taken to their GP, saying: 'You're busy, aren't you?'

My shift later that day was dominated by elderly patients. One woman, Doris, was brought in from a care home. Staff there hadn't been looking after her for long and now they were struggling with her aggression. I rang the manager of the care home to find out more. She told me Doris had advanced dementia which manifested in combative and volatile behaviour.

'I've tried everything to pacify her,' she said. 'Nothing works and I'm at my wits' end. We've had community teams out to assess her but they can't currently do anything because of the coronavirus situation. I'm sorry, I know A&E isn't the right place for her but I had no other choice.'

I put down the phone and went back to see Doris.

She was pleasant and I started to feed her yoghurt. A couple of seconds later she spat it out in my face. I tried again, but she bit on the spoon, yanked it from me and dropped it on the floor. It was 6 p.m. on a Sunday. There was no place for Doris to go apart from the hospital. I didn't really want to admit her but what choice did I have? I reluctantly picked up the phone and referred her to the hospital's healthcare of the elderly team. She was then taken up to the ward.

Dementia can be a vicious disease for both the person living with it and those around them. It steals memories and renders people unable to carry out day-to-day activities independently. It can be painful for those witnessing a loved one's decline as the person they thought they knew becomes someone completely different. That evening I saw three patients back to back with the condition.

One man refused to have anything covering his legs, which were spread wide open on the trolley, leaving absolutely nothing to the imagination. It's an almost daily occurrence that someone wants to show staff their tackle and people get more distressed if you try and afford them some modesty by putting a blanket over them. All that's left to do is to get on and treat them. They're usually oblivious to the situation.

Another woman appeared to be very lucid. She was pleasant, content and settled. I was having a normal conversation with her until she came out with: 'I'm living with my parents.' She was ninety. That was when

I saw the dementia. Some patients know where they are, what day it is, what year it is, while others think it's 1940. Sometimes I'll correct them but they usually look at me blankly. Other times, if I think it will cause more distress, I'll play along with what they're saying to a certain extent.

It had been difficult during the coronavirus outbreak so far because visitors weren't allowed into the hospital. Bringing someone with dementia into a hospital was already a disruption to their familiar surroundings and routine, and this could cause distress. At least before, it was possible for someone they knew to be there with them whether it was a care worker or a family member who could comfort them.

10

A Cry for Help

I came into work and found out I was to be on duty in one of the isolation units. The night shift team I took over from looked as though they had had an eventful time.

One of them said, 'I opened the curtain of a cubicle earlier to find my patient's girlfriend putting a tourniquet around his arm.'

'What?'

'Yeah, she was trying to find a vein in order to give him his daily hit of heroin.'

'How on earth did she sneak in?' I asked.

'No idea.'

I thought about it and wasn't surprised. This job has shown me the lengths people will go to when they're addicted to drugs or alcohol. Patients have stolen alcohol gel from the hand dispensers fixed to the walls in an attempt to satisfy cravings. I've also found patients smoking under the blanket.

People get up to all sorts when the curtains are closed. I've walked in on people having sex or carrying out other sexual acts. Call me a prude, but I firmly believe that A&E is not the place to be doing such things. I always tell them to stop and that it's inappropriate. I've seen other nurses in the same situation apologize and run off, embarrassed. I ask, 'What's going on?' They often reply, 'Oh, they're having an intimate moment.'

'Well, tell them to stop!' I say. I then barge in. 'Guys, can you stop it, please?'

I stand there until they cease any activity. Sometimes they're embarrassed, other times, they reply, 'Oh, I didn't have anything else to do.'

If you're having sex in A&E, I would argue that you don't need to be there so go and get a room. We had one man who came in a lot who we would always find masturbating. He'd stare at the curtain while he was doing it. I found it really creepy.

It was another hot day outside and I was hating wearing full PPE. After only having one isolation unit open, we were now back to using two. I didn't know if this was because Covid was on the rise or because people were increasingly feeling more relaxed about the pandemic and coming in with problems like chest pain that they had had for a while. I was in the middle of assessing someone and could feel the sweat running down my stomach, back, face and legs. It was everywhere and my chin felt drenched with moisture underneath my mask. It was distracting and I was starting to feel light-headed and seeing black spots in my vision. It was time to get out, sit down and drink copious amounts of water before I passed out and was no use to anyone.

I finished that shift and had the next couple of days at home recovering and preparing for a run of three nights. During my time off, I found myself consuming fiction and television series at an alarming rate. I had joined a book club, but sometimes struggled to keep up with it because of my work schedule. Ed and I met up a few times with another couple we're friendly with. Whenever I met up with non-NHS workers I was always reminded how our experiences of living through this pandemic were so different. They were generally stuck at home. I was still going to the hospital and coming home as normal, although I had learnt to appreciate the conversations I was having with my mum and sister. I'd also had more video chats with friends and I'd enjoyed those. I had made more of an effort to talk to people while before I'd stuff evenings with going out for dinner or to the cinema, choir and running club.

One of my friends had been furloughed. 'I'm finding it really difficult,' she told me when I saw her. 'I've tried to make an effort to keep some semblance of routine to my days but it's so hard. I have to be really strict with myself so I don't end up lounging in bed all day.' She also told me the experience had taught her who her real friends were and who she cared about. It was a time to re-evaluate the most important things in her life.

For me, I felt most of the things that mattered in my life – my work, my husband and my dogs – were firmly in place. I felt so lucky and privileged, though I did miss friends. I was also desperate to see my mum and sister. It wouldn't be long I kept telling myself, as we had arranged to meet halfway between where we were living for a socially distanced picnic in a couple of weeks' time.

The first of my run of night shifts in June was on a Friday. By this time, the number of daily deaths from Covid had dropped to around 350 and around 1,000 people in England were testing positive for the virus each day. One patient that evening was drunk when they came off their bike, another was drunk and hit by a van. One more was drunk when they fell off their child's scooter. After a couple of hours of her being in A&E while we carried out various investigations, I saw that she was very jittery and shaking hard. When someone shakes, it can be for a variety of reasons, but usually it's related to a surge in adrenalin, anxiety or pain. She'd had some strong painkillers so I thought it was something else.

I noticed that this woman had an uncontrollable tremor that had taken over her whole body. She couldn't do anything without dropping stuff or knocking objects over. She was also sweaty and looked bad. I thought it might be alcohol withdrawal.

'I know you've had an injury. There's also a mention of drinking on your charts. How much have you had?' I asked.

'Only a couple of glasses of wine,' she replied.

'Oh right? Do you drink much? How much do you have on a weekly basis, would you say?'

'I usually have a couple of glasses of wine, a couple of nights a week.'

She was lying. There was no way her shaking would be this bad if she was telling the truth. I wasn't in the mood to tiptoe round the subject so decided to go for the jugular. Withdrawal can be very dangerous as patients often have seizures, which can be fatal, so it was important that I found out what was going on.

'It looks to me like you're withdrawing from alcohol,' I said. 'I can give you medicine to help but I need to be sure it's alcohol withdrawal. If you're honest with me, I can help you.'

At that point, she became tearful. I realized she was probably using alcohol as a way of coping with something that had gone wrong and was painful.

'I drink two bottles of wine a day,' she admitted.

I didn't say anything more but gave her the appropriate medicine and left.

Normally, I'd do a bit of health promotion at this point, but I could tell she knew she had a problem and I didn't think me giving advice on how alcohol was harmful to health was appropriate at the time.

Often I'll ask how much a patient has to drink as part of my assessment. It surprises me how many people I come across that say they drink a couple of glasses of wine a night, every night. They say it out loud and then follow up with, 'I'm not an alcoholic.' I'll say, 'Do you think that might be a bit too much?' Regardless of whether they reply yes or no, I add, 'You should aim to have a couple of nights off alcohol a week if you can.'

They almost always come back with, 'I'm not an alcoholic, I don't drink a lot.'

'You're drinking every day and that's not good for you. You need to have a couple of nights off a week,' I'll reiterate.

To be honest, I don't think we're very good at health promotion in A&E. We're very busy and too task-focused. We have to work out if the person in front of us is dying. Do I need to bring them in? Can the GP follow up? Sometimes I'll do health promotion, but I often feel it falls on deaf ears. Maybe one patient will admit, 'I need to quit' and I'll tell them to go and see their GP and give them a leaflet about alcohol services or smoking cessation. I don't think I've ever had a patient say, 'Thank you. Oh yeah, I really do need to stop.' Usually, they'll say, 'Whatever. I'll keep doing what I want.' It's demoralizing when you can't see an end benefit.

With the woman I had seen that night, she was tired after having been up for hours. She needed to sleep. She knew she was in the wrong. She had lied and then opened up. Perhaps me pulling her up and making her confront what was happening was enough for now? I didn't want to add salt to the wound. Nevertheless, that didn't stop me from feeling a bit guilty at not doing more.

I was so busy that night that I was an hour late off shift. The roads were reasonably quiet, thankfully, so it was a quick drive home and straight to bed. I was wide awake three hours later and couldn't get back to sleep, no matter how hard I tried. I decided to go for a run. A woman who looked as though she was in her sixties saw me coming. I started veering off the path to give her a wide berth. She turned her back to me, head down, frozen to the spot like a statue. She seemed scared, and I don't think it was because of my red face. This wasn't the first time I'd had this type of encounter outside. I get hay fever and there's nothing less welcome than a person sneezing during a pandemic. There was one day when the pollen count was so high that I was sneezing continuously. Unfortunately I came across a man who could not have made it more obvious that he was terrified of me potentially spreading germs if he tried. I had already walked off the path and into the field and was a good five metres away from him but he practically threw himself into the hedge to get as far away from me as he could. Another time, I was approaching a gate with the dogs and a woman screamed 'STOP' and put her hand out. 'There's a sign on the gate that says someone with coronavirus might have touched it.'

'All right,' I replied.

'I just wanted to let you know. Do you need a hand

opening the gate?' She went to remove her scarf that she would use to avoid touching the gate.

'Oh don't worry. I'm OK, thanks.'

She was right, there was a handwritten note on the gate warning people of potential infection. The fear in some quarters was real.

I went into work and it wasn't long before a patient I had discharged a short while before, turned up again. 'I'm going to keep phoning for an ambulance until you admit me,' he said. Patients have served prison sentences for behaviour like this. And regular nuisance calls to emergency services have racked up bills amounting to thousands of pounds. Stories of people calling 999 for the wrong reason are common. I heard once that someone rang up complaining that their dog was unwell. Another time, someone asked for an ambulance then hung up. Paramedics arrived but the patient didn't want to be treated by someone with tattoos.

For some people with complex needs who often ring for an ambulance, care plans are put in place with involvement from teams across health and social care services. Despite everyone's efforts, for some patients the care they have is not enough and they continue to misuse ambulance services. I gave in to this man in the end and admitted him. I looked back through his A&E attendances and saw that I had seen him on previous occasions too.

After that rough start, I didn't know how I got through to the end of that shift with only one caffeinated drink and three hours' sleep. I felt surprisingly alert. The next day I spent mostly in bed trying to get as much rest as possible before my final night shift. I feel like I'm missing out if Ed does fun stuff without me, so he usually goes into night shift mode and refrains from going out too much. I appreciate the solidarity. Mum and my sister called for a chat. It emerged that my mum had been trying to encourage the start of a romantic liaison between my sister and the very few individuals she knew of who weren't over retirement age in the area. She had discovered that one was gay, which she seemed truly gutted about.

My final night shift was a mixed bag. I started off seeing a patient who was a prisoner. He was chatty and friendly. He'd come in with multiple skin abscesses and a couple were the size of grapefruits. We see quite a lot of prisoners in A&E but they only come in when things are really bad. Prisons have some healthcare facilities so if they've ended up with us, it's usually because something's really wrong.

They, along with the prison guards, always call me 'Miss' which I find a bit weird because it makes me feel like a teacher. I rarely know what they've done to end up behind bars and I don't ask, it's not necessary. I see them as patients who need treating. They've got medical problems and it's my job to try and sort them out.

I can usually have a guess at what they're locked up for depending on which prison they've come in from.

There's one for sex offenders in the area, for example. I can also tell the severity of their crimes by the length of the chain attaching them to prison guards as well as the type of handcuffs they've got on. If the chain is long and the handcuffs look flimsy, they're not that dangerous. Once I had a patient who had a swollen wrist and I didn't know if it was a fracture. I couldn't assess his wrist properly because of the thick handcuffs he had on that were so tight that he couldn't move his hands apart at all. I asked the prison guard, 'Can we remove these please?' Sometimes they'll take one off, but on that occasion, I was told a firm 'no'. He had obviously done something very wrong and was still dangerous. Everyone has a right to treatment, though, and I will give it, no matter what.

I started work on my latest prisoner patient and was waiting for some tests to come back when I had to step away for a meeting with colleagues in an adjacent office to discuss some aspects of patient care. I'd seen and heard some commotion earlier, when the police brought in a man who had been assaulted. He'd started yelling at some staff.

'That's enough of that,' said one police officer. 'Don't talk to the staff like that when they're going to help you. You need to apologize.'

'Sorry,' grumbled the man, very half-heartedly.

The police officer turned to the nurses and said, 'Right, we'll leave him with you. We've got to get a move on.'

They left because the man they had brought in wasn't under arrest. Within seconds, all hell broke loose. He crashed into the room where I was sitting and started mouthing off. I decided to confront him.

'Excuse me, you can't come in here because we are having confidential discussions about patients,' I said.

'Fuck you, I've been assaulted,' he replied.

'Yes, I can see that, but you telling me doesn't make it any more dramatic.'

'I need stitching.'

'Fine, but currently with the way you're behaving, that's not going to happen.'

At that point, he saw red. The situation escalated rapidly. He started spitting in my face and calling me 'a fucking cunt'. I stood my ground.

'At the moment, with the way you're behaving you may as well leave, because no one will care for you in this state,' I continued. 'If you calm down, we're more than happy to help you.'

If the worst happened and he punched me, at least I was already in hospital. There were also plenty of witnesses. I heard another patient start to cry, saying, 'I'm scared.' One of the registrars came into the room and told me to get out. I stayed where I was. I didn't see how it was any better if the registrar was punched instead of me. Four burly security guards then appeared. They tried to calm him down but it wasn't working. The man's fists were clenched, his eyes were wide open and his pupils dilated, he was in fight mode. By this time, blood was leaking from him all over the place. In his anger, he'd torn open one of his wounds which had dried and clotted over. The scene was one of carnage. The police then arrived a few minutes later and arrested him. I wondered what makes someone so angry and full of hate. How did he get like that?

I returned to my prisoner patient. He had heard all the commotion. Who hadn't? 'What a dick,' he said. Yep, I thought, but I didn't pass comment. I'm certainly not a fan of the c-word but I find it quite easy to brush those sorts of comments off. They don't feel that personal and I know that swearing at someone in a situation like that is completely unreasonable. What really gets to me is when patients or relatives get angry because they're not happy with the care that's been provided. I feel guilty in those situations, replaying every moment over and over in my mind, wishing I'd done things differently even though logically I know I did my best.

For the rest of the shift, all I saw were people with mental health problems. It had been the same the night before when my team in majors saw at least three people who had attempted suicide, and a couple had to be intubated to keep them breathing. Meanwhile, colleagues in minors had seen a raft of patients with anxiety.

There were patients who had self-harmed, taken overdoses, or were in depressive or anxious states. Every single one mentioned the virus as a contributing factor.

I must have heard 'since lockdown' over a hundred times. Patients had started smoking since lockdown, alcohol consumption had gone up since lockdown, financial worries had rocketed since lockdown, relationships had become more strained since lockdown. Nobody could get a break and situations had reached boiling point.

It was startling how many serious mental health episodes we were having to deal with in people who had no history of any problems. It was a continuation of what we had seen earlier in the crisis, but now it seemed worse. People had been dealing with restrictions on everyday life for coming up to three months. More than 40,000 people in the UK had died from coronavirus. All this was having an impact. It became somewhat routine to me, as awful as that sounds. I had to consciously remind myself that a first-time suicide attempt was a huge event in someone's life, even if I'd seen it so many times before. One patient disclosed such an attempt to me, expecting a huge reaction, but it was the tenth one I'd seen in the past few days. And a lot of my focus is on the medical side of things rather than their emotional needs. What had they taken, would there be any nasty side-effects, what blood tests did I need to do, did I need to admit them? It was a mechanical way of doing things but this was what A&E and I needed to make sure they didn't die. Despite that, I always remembered that it was my role as a nurse to make sure I listened to patients if they wanted, or needed, to tell me something.

There was one man who had come in after an attempt to take his own life who told me he had a daughter with cerebral palsy.

'I'm a single dad and have been struggling more than ever since lockdown.'

'Have you tried asking social services for more help for your child?' I asked.

'Yes, they told me there was nothing they could do.'

I could see he was getting no respite and was at the end of his tether.

'Now because of lockdown I don't have a break. She's not at school and I've lost my job. I can't go out,' he added.

'You're doing a great job,' I told him. 'I can't imagine how hard it is for you. Your daughter needs you. What would she do if you were gone?'

'There'd be a better parent out there for her,' he added.

I felt so sad but was also aware that I had to fill out a load of paperwork to make sure the daughter was safe. Often it's not just the patient you have to think of, but those around them that rely on them.

Next up was a young patient who was a victim of domestic abuse. Earlier that night, she had been thrown to the ground, held down with her face pushed down so hard that she had carpet burns. Her partner had stubbed countless cigarettes out all over her back. The police had been called by a neighbour who had heard shouting and screaming. I was horrified, but relieved that she had escaped and that we could now protect her. I woke up various on-call support workers, ringing round in an attempt to find her an emergency bed in a refuge. There were none, so she came into hospital until we could find her somewhere safe to go.

I finished my shift after seeing her off to the ward. It had been a devastating set of nights, but nothing out of the ordinary for A&E. Only three more shifts to go until I had a week's break, but of course they weren't going to be easy.

11

Time for a Break

I was counting down the hours to the start of my annual leave as I began a shift in the isolation unit. The temperature had dropped significantly so wearing PPE was much more bearable. I saw an elderly man who had been sent to A&E by a healthcare worker who visited him at home. They thought he had sepsis. Sepsis is terrifying for those that work in healthcare because it can be easy to miss and there have been cases where people have died because of errors. It is the body's response to an infection and can cause a patient to go into multiple organ failure. Not only is death a real possibility, but survivors can be left with the devastating lifelong effects of the illness. It's important to treat it as quickly as possible to avoid these. There's loads of data that shows that every hour that passes without treatment, someone's chances of dying or developing complications rise.

We have a team within the hospital dedicated to educating staff around sepsis so that we can recognize it quickly and take effective action. It has become a big thing in the last year or two because of the impact sepsis can have. I underwent a day's training where former patients came in to talk to staff about post sepsis syndrome, which is where someone has difficulty sleeping and can suffer nightmares, panic attacks, difficulty concentrating as well as a loss of self-esteem and depression. One man did a talk about the importance of recognizing it quickly and spoke about his struggles. Others said they'd lost loved ones. They were a visual reminder for us to always think about sepsis. I sat there feeling devastated. I felt personally responsible, even though I knew I wasn't. I wanted to stand up and say 'I'm sorry.' They'd been through so much but were strong enough to come back and talk about their experiences so we could do better.

So now I went down our sepsis checklist, which has markers to look for to see if a patient might have it. He had a high temperature but his blood pressure was on the low side and his heart was trying to compensate by pumping faster. He had lost his sense of taste and had abdominal pain. He had the symptoms of Covid-19 but as I progressed in my examination, I felt a mass in his abdomen. It was the size of my two fists put together and was tender. He needed an abdominal scan, but in my role as an ACP, I couldn't request one so I had to go and ask a senior colleague to approve it.

As the role of an ACP is still quite new, we often face inequalities when it comes to what we can do compared to a doctor. The speciality of radiology for example insists that a chunk of imaging can still only be requested by those who have qualified as a doctor. I could work in A&E for twenty years as an ACP and not be able to request something vital to carrying out my job, while a junior doctor fresh out of university who has just qualified and worked for a couple of days in the department is taken more seriously in some quarters.

I once referred a patient and the speciality consultant said they wanted to talk to my registrar. I went to get him and he said exactly the same thing as me. Perhaps they didn't take me seriously because I wasn't assertive enough, or perhaps it was because my title wasn't 'Dr'. Patients can be just the same though. There have been times when I've gone to tell a patient they can go home with some advice on what to do about their condition only to hear them demand, 'I want to speak to the doctor.' The doctor comes along and repeats what I've just said. The patient dutifully listens and obeys.

It's frustrating, it's rude, it's hurtful and it's demoralizing. I've been doing this job for years. Some nurses have been in A&E for decades and have so much experience and exposure that they can tell what's wrong with a patient just by looking at them.

Since I started my career, the hierarchy has flattened out a lot and there's more of an appreciation that nurses are up-skilling and becoming autonomous decision-makers. One positive thing about the pandemic was that it had raised the profile of nursing. The general public definitely had more of an appreciation of us, but even so many still thought we were there to do bed baths and wipe bottoms. Nurses, and female healthcare professionals in general, have a tough time smashing patriarchal views and outdated stereotypes that are still present.

I went to find a doctor, explained my patient's situation to him and asked if he would request a scan for me.

'I don't think that's necessary,' he told me.

'I think it is,' I replied. 'There's a definite tender mass in his abdomen that I think needs investigating today.'

'No, we've got enough to worry about. Send them home for the GP to arrange a scan.'

'I really think we should do a scan.'

Eventually he agreed. I was so relieved, especially when the scan revealed there was something there. The radiologist couldn't determine whether it was a cancer of some kind or an appendicitis that had engulfed the bowel. Either way, it was serious. This was probably the source of my patient's temperature, but he could be doubly unfortunate and also have the virus.

I went back and told him: 'Your scan has shown that there is a mass in your tummy. We're not totally sure what it is, so you need to come into hospital so the surgeons can take you to theatre and have a closer look.'

He looked at me blankly. I was not sure he had taken everything in. Was he confused? I didn't want to cause more distress, so if he hadn't grasped the full extent of what I had said, there was no point in banging on about it.

Unlike back in April when the hospital had three isolation units going but ample staff to run them, the amount of people on shift had decreased as the numbers of people with coronavirus had fallen. We were now starting off with one isolation unit open in the morning. By lunch, it might have filled up and another one would have to open in the afternoon. On those days, I was rushed off my feet. Eight people would come in all at once and there'd be a flurry of activity with me making decisions and plans for existing patients while trying to care for the new ones. What was worse was that some people were turning up really sick, much more so than a month or so before. I didn't know why. Were they delaying asking for help? Did they think we were still in the thick of it and didn't want to bother us?

In complete contrast, when I was away from work, it seemed like people had forgotten about the pandemic we were embroiled in and that was absolutely not over. Numbers had decreased but there were still hundreds of people dying a day. Only a few shifts before, I had a call from someone working in the intensive care unit asking if a patient's wedding ring had been left in A&E. By the time we found it half an hour later, they had died. I knew lockdown was boring and challenging but I was tired of hearing about and seeing deaths that could have been avoided.

What really stood out to me was seeing the queue for McDonald's. I couldn't get into the retail outlet to go to the supermarket because the roads were blocked. I didn't even understand what was so great about eating the food produced there. I'm well aware how controversial that opinion is, as when I told some colleagues I'd never had a burger from McDonald's they looked at me with such disdain.

The people coming in to the isolation unit now and testing positive for Covid-19 must have caught the virus during lockdown. Their shock at how this could have happened never failed to surprise me.

'You've got the virus,' I'd tell them.

'Oh, I don't know how that's happened,' they'd say. 'I've been locked down for the past couple of weeks.'

'Have you left the house?'

'Yes.'

'Have you had contact with other people?'

'Yes, my relative comes round every day to see if I'm OK and do any odd jobs around the house.'

'That's probably why then. You've got this from your socializing or from your relative.'

I was flabbergasted at some people's ignorance around how viruses spread. I sometimes wished it was visible, like the emoji of a neon green splodge, because then the public's approach to it would be different. Perhaps people would think twice about touching a door that various people had access to and then not washing their hands afterwards. It was really difficult not to get frustrated, especially when I knew people were not adhering to lockdown as they should have been.

One colleague told me that they had got home after a day at work only to find their partner and children not there. They'd phoned the partner who said they were round at a neighbour's house because it was a sunny day. My colleague went round to find all the children playing with each other and having a party. It was soul-destroying for that nurse who had just spent twelve hours looking after Covid patients to come home to their own family disobeying the rules. And I heard variations on this story from other staff. People's interpretations of the rules were so different. In some cases, it seemed that unless individuals were personally affected by a relative who had died, they thought they were invincible and had little regard for the lives of others.

The next day, I was working in resus when I was called to see a patient in supraventricular tachycardia – a very fast heart rhythm, which if left untreated can be fatal. The symptoms are palpitations or feeling short of breath. The only way to treat it is with a drug that switches the patient's heart back into its normal rhythm. This isn't any old drug, however, and administering it is terrifying both for the patient and the healthcare professional.

'You've got an irregular heartbeat,' I told my patient. 'To fix it, I'm going to give you this drug. It works rapidly, usually within a few seconds. It will make you feel as though your heart is stopping. It will give you a sense of impending doom and make you feel as though you might die. It will make you feel like you're falling but we're here and you need this to make you feel better.'

He looked at me aghast, but realized that I needed to get a move on. I injected the dose very quickly into a large cannula that we'd inserted as close to the heart as possible and flushed it down with saline to get it moving. My consultant was with me, so if something went wrong we were all in safe hands.

Within a few seconds, the look of nervousness on my patient's face turned to panic, and tears appeared in his eyes before he started groaning and losing consciousness. I held his hand saying, 'It's going to be OK, we've got you.' I kept looking at the defibrillator, where I saw his heart rate plummet from 180 beats per minute to zero. The line across the screen was slightly wavy (the flat line you see in movies is not real) instead of jagged; my patient's heart was stopping.

Normally at this point, I would have started doing compressions but in this case I had to stand, watch and wait for what felt like hours, but in reality was a couple of seconds.

'It's working,' I said to my patient.

If he stayed like this for a couple of seconds longer, he would be in cardiac arrest and I'd have to start trying to revive him. I waited with bated breath until

I saw his heartbeat resume on the screen. I think in that moment I was more relieved than my patient. When he came round, he said, 'Oh I feel great. Thank you! Can I go home now?'

This time it was a success, but sometimes it doesn't work first time so you have to give an increased dose. The whole process is repeated. The patient dreads it because they've got to go through the motions of dying all over again. From a healthcare professional's point of view, the fear also looms large. This procedure is always so intense and any clinician who says they don't feel anxious when they watch the heart rate and rhythm on the defibrillator is lying. There have been times when the heart stops for a beat too long and everybody in the room has started thinking about jumping into action, before it starts again. We have to mask our worries though, because it's imperative that we're supportive for the patient, even when deep down we are petrified ourselves.

My sense of calm and relief didn't last long as I was alerted to a patient who had arrived with two fingers missing.

'All right, love!' he said cheerfully as I appeared before him. 'Any chance of a cup of tea?'

He was in remarkably good spirits for someone who had just lost their fingers.

'What's happened to you, then?' I asked.

'I cut my fingers off with a circular saw while doing some home renovations.'

His hand was heavily bandaged but there must have been so much blood at the scene when the paramedics arrived, not that you'd know it from this guy, who was pretty tough and not fazed in the slightest.

'My fingers are following in a bag of vegetables,' he added. 'It was the only frozen thing I could find to keep them cool.'

We're used to body parts in A&E. Lots of people use circular saws and Stanley knives so there's plenty of opportunity for things to go wrong. I've treated a patient who managed to take their arm off at the elbow. It's a bit bizarre when somebody comes in afterwards carrying the rest of the patient who is before you. There's very little that A&E does in these situations, unless the patient needs resuscitating or a transfusion. This guy was sitting up and was chatting away. His bleeding had been controlled. The fingers arrived, but I did not go digging around for them among the frozen peas and carrots. This was a job for the surgeons. I phoned them and said goodbye to my patient as he was taken off to theatre. It was time to eat. Nothing puts me off my food.

After lunch, a patient was rushed in with anaphylaxis. She'd had a Chinese takeaway and had a nut allergy so we assumed there might have been some nuts within what she had eaten. She had used her epi-pen to no effect. The ambulance crew had given her a further two doses of adrenalin and she was still having difficulty breathing. She had passed the point of rapid breathing in a desperate attempt to get more oxygen to her lungs and was tiring. It wasn't long before she resorted to abdominal breathing which occurs when the body is trying everything it can to get air in and out. She was taking about five or six breaths a minute, which was nowhere near enough. Her airway was closing up and if we didn't intubate her soon, there would be no room for us to pass a tube down. We called for an anaesthetist and threw all the medications we could at her while they took the lift down three floors to get to A&E.

Intubation is a difficult procedure. Only certain consultants in A&E are trained to do it and it's not something they do regularly. When you've got an anaesthetist on hand, they are always the first port of call. Anaesthetists are pretty high up the healthcare food chain and get paid a lot, but they're worth it. They are responsible for the airway. Nothing else happens if the airway is compromised, it's the most important thing.

The anaesthetist that day came strolling in and slickly did what needed to be done. It looked as easy as pouring a cup of tea. He then left while the rest of us looked on in awe before sending the patient up to intensive care. I have been in the room on a couple of occasions where an anaesthetist has really struggled. You see the sweat on their collar when they're trying to manage a difficult intubation. Perhaps the airway is so swollen nothing will fit, or there's something lodged in there. Sometimes an airway is so deformed after a trauma, or there's loads of blood everywhere which makes it very stressful for them. They know everybody is watching and that their one and only job in the situation is to stick a tube down someone's throat. If that can't happen that's it, the patient will die.

The red phone on the wall in the middle of resus alerted us to our next patient. A man had been pulled out of the canal and was on his way to us. He was in cardiac arrest and had a body temperature of 27°C. A normal temperature is about 36°C. He had hypothermia and when he arrived he was quickly transferred onto a Lucas machine, which can perform cardiac compressions. He needed resuscitation over a long period and as humans tire quickly, the quality of compressions gets worse.

The repetitive, mechanical noise of a Lucas machine is one recognized by any A&E staff member. It's a really aggressive machine which consists of a massive suction cup that is thrust down and punches a patient's chest. What makes it worse for me is that the patient's arms are strapped onto it so they look like they are hugging it. I know its purpose is to give good, effective, potentially life-saving compressions, but to see such a horrible and loud machine embraced by a dying patient is disturbing and bizarre to look at. I find it really difficult.

We've had lots of people who have been fished out of the canal turn up in the department. Quite a lot of homeless people camp beside it and sometimes fall in. Cyclists and joggers also fall in. Drowning is a very real danger, and people often don't realize that there doesn't need to be a lot of water for someone to die. It only takes a couple of centimetres of water to cover the airway. I always remember the story my dad used to tell about one of his uncles trying to drown him in the bath when he was a child. It was so memorable because he'd suddenly announce with a deadpan expression: 'My uncle tried to drown me in the bath when I was a child.' Everyone around him was shocked and after a short silence asked, 'Why? What happened next?' to which he would reply, 'I don't remember.' Any efforts to get more information were futile.

After an hour, the team decided to stop the Lucas machine from attempting resuscitation. We didn't know who our patient was. I guessed he might have been in his thirties, but I didn't know. While his identity remained a mystery, we had given him a name from the phonetic alphabet like Foxtrot Tango. We used to call patients 'unknown' if we didn't know their identity and if there was more than one in a shift, they would be unknown 2, 3, 4 and so on. Once we had five unknowns in over the course of a night. We would also give them a date of birth that made them 110 years old to remind you that your patient wasn't actually called Foxtrot Tango.

Had this man fallen into the canal, was he pushed or had he killed himself? The police had turned up to try and find out who he was and whether he had any family.

The police often have our back. We used to have

them patrol the department, and there'd be a specific office set aside for them. Now because of cuts to the force, they can't offer that service, and we're largely left to fend for ourselves.

There are single members of staff who make more of an effort with some of the police officers. I suppose they're a new face and a potential romantic prospect. When you work unsociable hours, it's difficult to find the time to meet a partner and form a relationship elsewhere. There are four people I know who are in relationships with police officers and they all met through work.

A&E, weirdly, is a hotbed of desire. Countless relationships are formed in the department. Unfortunately, many have also ended and the tension can be cut with a knife. The only constant is that people always find out about everything. You cannot keep a secret in A&E.

A lot of the consultants are married to anaesthetists or occupational therapists or other doctors within A&E and across the hospital. Romance is rife. I'd go so far as to say that if you've not cemented a relationship before starting work in A&E, you're guaranteed to fall in love on the job.

There are a deal of positives associated with going out with someone who works in healthcare. I often get frustrated with my husband; sometimes he'll ask how my day was, but he doesn't understand half of what I go through and he never will. Likewise, I will never know what goes on in his job. Sometimes that is difficult because I can't emotionally offload onto him. Someone working in healthcare will know what you mean and how you're feeling after you say a couple of words, sometimes. But then when you're in a relationship with another healthcare professional, you never really get away from work and sometimes Ed can provide a different perspective. There are arguments both ways.

On my final shift before a week off, I was in isolation again. An elderly patient arrived who was very frail indeed. His blood pressure was so low that it was unrecordable and his oxygen saturations were at 56 per cent when the ambulance crew arrived at his care home. He looked as pale as the white bed sheet he was lying on. He was going to die. The care home was informing the family, but otherwise he was on his own. We made him comfortable, brushed his hair, mopped his forehead and held a wet sponge to his lips and then made plans for him to be transferred up to one of the wards so he could be in a more peaceful environment. One of the staff members up there would be free to take time to be with him in his final moments.

Seconds later, seven patients arrived all at once. They all looked terrible. These were more people that had held out at home and come to us in A&E later than we would have liked. There were only three clinicians on the unit, including me, so we quickly darted from patient to patient, ordering investigations and getting the ball rolling with their treatment. I got to a good point and sat down to write my patient's notes up when one of my nursing colleagues tapped me on the shoulder.

'Louise, do you know when someone will be available to see the next patient?'

'It surely can't be me. I've just seen a patient and am already rushed off my feet.'

'I think someone needs to see this patient as soon as possible,' she continued. 'She looks unwell.'

'How unwell are we talking?' I asked, desperately trying to input my notes into the computer system while simultaneously trying to order various tests.

'Just turn around, Louise.'

I did so reluctantly because I really wanted to get one job finished without being interrupted so I could move on to the next.

'Oh my God! She's trying to die.'

My notes had to wait. I rushed over.

'Get the defibrillator pads on her, she looks like she's about to arrest,' I told my colleague.

A woman lay before me, hardly breathing. I looked at her notes. She was only in her fifties. She was apparently fine yesterday, but started with 'a bit of a cough' in the evening. Her blood gas showed she was in respiratory failure. I got flashbacks to when Shirley deteriorated in the space of fifteen minutes in my care and I had to send her to intensive care to be intubated. She had survived, but would I be as lucky a second time? Fears of not being competent or confident enough flooded my mind again. I started to panic. I'd just seen another patient who was sick and dying. This one was about to arrest. I felt so overwhelmed.

I reminded myself to go back to basics. A for airway. My patient was hardly breathing and I couldn't do much about it, so it was time to call intensive care. I read out the gas result and that was enough to send them on their way down. They knew we couldn't have patients in the department a second longer than they needed to be because of the threat of overcrowding and the need to keep everyone socially distanced. They swooped in and took the patient away to be intubated. I sat back down to finish my notes.

Another patient's X-ray came back looking like he had Covid-19. He needed oxygen. I rang his next of kin, his son, to discuss the possibility of a DNAR because he was frail and elderly with a whole host of other health problems.

It was difficult to have these sorts of conversations over the phone. I hadn't had to have many like this up until this point as it was usually left up to my colleagues on the wards who had more time to talk to people and explain everything. Over the phone, I couldn't see the person I was talking to or read their eyes and body language. Patients' relatives get understandably anxious. People are worried about A&E as it is, it has life or death connotations that make people panic. On top of that, there was the pandemic, and people couldn't see their loved ones in hospital.

This relative was angry. He'd taken his father into

hospital for an unrelated issue a few weeks before. It appeared as though he had caught the virus either there or in the interim. First I had to diffuse that anger. I could empathize with his situation and so managed to bring him down from boiling to a point where I could explain what was happening. Then I had to drop the bombshell that we wouldn't be attempting resuscitation on his father. Luckily he was understanding and open to the discussion. It was still ridiculously hard to have this conversation over the phone, though.

Although it went well, I was all too aware it could have gone very differently. I was also reminded of how many more DNARs we had been filling out since the pandemic had begun. The chances of recovering from Covid when someone was elderly were very slim and it was so important to keep the family in the loop and involved at every step of their care, even if we had to do it over the phone. In some cases, the person didn't have any family and so they were alone.

At that moment, I suddenly felt a pang of sympathy for my colleagues in intensive care and on the wards. There have always been people who have died alone, but there were so many more at the moment. Those who were end-of-life were granted permission to have one visitor but some relatives didn't want to come into hospital for fear of catching the virus and because they were also vulnerable. I could understand as although they would be in full PPE, they didn't have the training or the experience that we had undergone in order to learn about how to put it on and take it off properly.

It was often left to the nurses to sit with patients for hours while they died and they were doing this more than normal. People enter the nursing profession to help, cure and make people better. Of course, death is a part of the job, but no one wants to deal with it day in, day out.

I'd been so busy that I'd hardly had time to follow up on another patient who had turned up with all the others. 'I've been feeling intermittently short of breath for the past three months,' she told me when I first saw her.

'And how have you been affected? Would you be able to tell me what impact your breathlessness has had on your daily life please?'

'Oh, it hasn't stopped me from doing anything. It hasn't really bothered me to be honest.'

'OK, and what are you hoping to get from us in A&E today?'

'I just thought I'd come to get checked out.'

I had sent her off for a chest X-ray, which had come back looking fine. Amid all the chaos, she had told one of my nursing colleagues that she wanted to leave. That was fine by me. I told my colleague to give her the appropriate advice on when to come back. I wondered whether seeing and hearing all the commotion had put her situation into perspective.

My next patient had suddenly become short of breath that morning and had woken up because of it. I listened to his chest and ordered a chest X-ray, which confirmed he had a pneumothorax. This, and not Covid, was the reason for his breathlessness, so I sent him to the cold area for colleagues there to insert a chest drain.

By this time, I'd been in PPE for seven and a half hours with no drink or toilet break. I was painfully aware that I needed to stop doing this. I escaped for a break and knew that in just a couple of hours I would be able to leave work behind me, or at least try, and embark on my annual leave. I was meant to have gone to a festival in the Netherlands with my husband. Not only was that cancelled, but the weather had taken a turn for the worse. Gone was the glorious sunshine. Instead, the forecast said we were in for a week of showers. At least I'd be able to crack on with my dissertation and start *Game of Thrones*.

12

Bad Dreams

I woke up the next morning and felt relief that I wouldn't be going into hospital for another week. Ed had time off too and we decided to go slightly further afield when walking the dogs. On one day trip to the coast we even saw some blue skies. More often than not, though, we were kitted out in full waterproofs and walked through the rain while getting increasingly hot and sweaty. It wasn't far away from the feeling of wearing PPE but we still returned home wet and muddy.

The weather was unrelenting and I couldn't help but feel I was missing out because this was not the holiday I had planned. I caught up with friends – at a distance – and even met one by the river, where we sat drinking cans of gin and tonic in pouring rain. Thankfully the forecast for Saturday, the day set aside for my family reunion, looked promising.

Seeing my mum and sister for the first time since my father's funeral in February was lovely and emotional all at the same time. Mum looked like she'd lost weight. I wanted to give them both a hug, but didn't. I also wanted to go and spend time with them at the house where I had grown up and still call home. Of course, I wasn't allowed to do that either so a picnic in a woodland area halfway between where we both lived had to suffice.

The sun came out and we went on a walk through the trees. It wasn't long until, for some light relief, we found a way to segue into stories of my sister's eccentricities. Mum had started to flag just before the end of the walk and discussion turned to my sister's strops when she felt she had walked too far and didn't want to go on any longer.

The first time she met one of my brothers-in-law, we did Parkrun, which she did not enjoy, before going on a walk that he had chosen. She thought it was going to be a gentle stroll for a couple of hours at most, and that black skinny jeans and a pair of flimsy trainers would therefore be appropriate. Four hours after we started walking, we were in the middle of nowhere with no signs of civilization in sight. We had hiked up steep hills, climbed over rocks, leapt over streams and clambered over undulating landscape.

My sister had reached her limit and things weren't helped when every time she asked how long was left, she was told the same amount of time. She threw the most almighty strop. To be honest, I was feeling the same but she has always been more forthright and vocal with her opinions.

'I don't mind doing long walks, but you should have told me before so I could mentally prepare!' she yelled in frustration. 'You have to manage my expectations!'

She hadn't brought any water or snacks and I didn't have any to appease her either. We ended up walking at least ten miles that day before we sat down in a pub.

'I'm not walking any more,' she announced.

'Errr, the car's not here,' I replied.

'I don't care! I'm not moving.'

Ed ended up running to get the car to bring it to her. After re-telling this story, we moved on to the time the three of us met up at Glastonbury. It was my sister's first time at the festival and she and my husband set about demolishing a bottle of gin. It tipped it down so hard with rain that the main stage closed. We remained in the middle of a field sheltering under an umbrella. When the deluge eased, the music started again and Ed fell asleep on a stranger's shoulder while my sister wailed; the gin had got to her. We were camping in neighbouring fields so when it came to making our way back to our tents, Ed kept falling asleep on his feet but somehow seemed to know exactly where he was going. Meanwhile, the enormous amount of mud got the better of my sister and she threw another strop. After slipping for the umpteenth time, she stood still where she was and cried out: 'I can't do this anymore! I'm tired, my feet hurt so much. This is NOT enjoyable.' I stood there laughing at her standing deep in mud, while Ed went to give her a helping hand.

'I'm glad I wasn't there,' said my mother.

*   *   *

After a week off, I should have felt refreshed, energized and eager to return to work. I didn't. Normally when Ed and I have time off, we spend it far from home doing exciting activities or exploring new places. I felt like I hadn't had a great time and that it had gone by too quickly. I didn't feel rested either because I still hadn't been sleeping well. My dreams had got worse and were now filled with images of past patients.

I saw the faces of some of the really sick people I'd treated who had died. They'd been on their way out of this world for a while and their skin was white and waxy, sometimes with a yellow tinge. Their faces were really drawn with a sunken mouth and eyes. If it was an old person and they didn't have any dentures in, there was no shape to the bottom of their mouth so it gaped open.

Occasionally, I was haunted by the patient who had died from a gastrointestinal bleed, hosing out blood from every orifice, but more often than not it was the face of someone who was dying slowly that invaded my subconscious over and over again.

Whenever I meet someone and tell them what I do for a living, one of the first questions they always ask is: 'What's the worst thing you've ever seen?' I get it from hairdressers, the in-laws, friends of friends, my husband's work colleagues on a night out and loads more people. The conversation usually starts with: 'I bet you've seen some things.' Silence follows while I work out what to say. I think about how long I have to engage with this person. Will it be a brief encounter or will I be stuck with them for a few hours or more? If it's the latter, I might tell them a gory story – like the teenager who got impaled by a fence but was ultimately fine because their injuries were quite an easy thing for us to deal with. People want drama and a happy ending. No one wants to hear about the young man who was out on his motorbike and crashed, killing his friend who was riding on the back without a helmet on, or the baby who was mauled to death by a dog. Those types of stories are conversation stoppers. I made the mistake once of opening up about what I'd seen to someone I'd just met. They went quiet. 'Oh God,' they said and that was it.

'That's my job! That's what I do,' I replied jokily after the silence became too awkward to bear.

Would conversations now start with: 'What was it like working through the pandemic?' It was already beginning to happen. In a shop in town the woman behind the counter asked, 'How has it been?'

It's funny because sometimes I'll come home and tell Ed about a dramatic episode at work and he'll exaggerate it and go and tell his colleagues over lunch and get a huge reaction. He'll never mention how I had to hold an old lady's hand while she died because she was on her own, though, or the person who killed themselves. Those stories are too sad for office chat and yet they are the cases that hit me the hardest.

I'd had one dream in particular a couple of times.

I saw my dad on the floor against the chair where he died. I wasn't there when he passed away but Mum had told us the details and I could picture it clearly because I've been in A&E when someone's died after vomiting blood. In my dream, I could see the blood, it was congealed – and I could smell it. It was like I was stood over Dad unable to do anything. Once, I woke up halfway through the dream with tears running down my cheeks. My husband had also woken up and said I'd been whimpering and sounded like one of the dogs.

'Are you all right?' he asked.

'Yeah, yeah. Fine.'

He fell asleep again while I lay there thinking and recovering from the horror. I couldn't imagine how my mum was coping after witnessing him die like that. I must have managed to drift off again because the next thing I knew the alarm was ringing and I had to get up for work.

I'd heard that lots of people were having weird and vivid dreams during lockdown. I was no different. Work was on my mind more than ever and I didn't have my normal life to distract me. It was becoming painfully clear that my way of dealing with the trauma I see at work was not adequate and that I needed to look after myself a bit more. I was beginning to realize that I needed to become more aware of how the job was affecting me. A lot of the time, those of us who work in A&E will just brush something off; we think we're tough because we see awful stuff all the time. When we're at work, we just carry on. But now that memories were penetrating my subconscious and affecting my sleep, I knew I needed to start looking after my mental health more. The next day I found out that there were plans to develop a longer-term staff support and well-being plan in the department. This was something positive to come from the pandemic.

I walked into hospital in the morning sweaty after my overdressed cycle ride. While I'd been off the third isolation unit had been dismantled and was being used for normal A&E patients. Hospital guidelines had also changed and now stated that everyone should wear a face mask in all areas. A bleary-eyed volunteer was holding a box of face masks for everyone who walked through the doors. I wondered what time she had started, considering that I was walking in at 6.30 a.m.

Our regular volunteers had stopped working during the coronavirus crisis. We usually have one woman, Sally, who makes cups of tea for patients and offers them food. Then there's another man, Geoff, who is simply fabulous. When I used to triage patients, I'd bring them out and he'd be there ready to take them to where they needed to go. Geoff had been massively missed but he was in the at-risk category. He had been receiving treatment for cancer. We were all so sad when he was diagnosed but he still came to work. 'As long as I've got the energy, I'll still come,' he said. They are both much-loved members of A&E.

There was another man who delivered newspapers and went round with a trolley packed with sweets and chocolate, cracking the same jokes as he went. He reminded me a bit of Dad with his quips that always made everyone laugh. Another very popular volunteer was the man who came in with two therapy dogs for the staff and patients.

We've got a Facebook group for everyone who works at the trust and he had posted 'I'm missing you guys' on it. There were hundreds of comments below asking him to bring the dogs in, so he posted a picture of one of them wearing a surgical mask. We'd all noticed the volunteers' absence and I hoped we could get them back in the department soon.

Later that day I was working on a patient when I overheard a conversation between a man and one of the junior nurses. I couldn't make out exactly what was being said but it seemed heated. His voice was getting louder and louder. I left it for a while until it was clear the nurse was starting to struggle and he was stopping her from being able to get on with her job. A lot of the newer nurses are softer than those of us who have been in A&E for a while. I used to be like that too but after eight years I've grown a thicker skin and my tolerance for bullshit is low.

'What's the problem here?' I asked, seeing a wave of relief cross the nurse's face at my intervention.

'This nurse can't seem to give me a good reason why I should have to wear a mask,' the man shouted, spitting saliva from the corners of his mouth. He looked angry, with a red face and distended veins.

'It's hospital policy that everyone now wears a face mask both for their own protection and for that of everyone else. We are still in the middle of a pandemic,' I replied.

'Well I don't have the virus, so what's the point?' he retorted.

'Unfortunately you can't be sure you don't have the virus unless you've been tested very recently. You could be asymptomatic. We have vulnerable patients all around you and it's important that we try to protect everyone during this public health crisis.'

The conversation went on like this until I saw that I wasn't going to get anywhere. The man was becoming more agitated and taking up too much of my nursing colleague's and my time. I had five patients on the go and needed to get back to review one who had deteriorated.

'It's up to you, sir. We can only do our best to protect our patients, but we can't force you to do anything.'

With that, the nurse and I left him with no one to have a go at. He stood there puzzled for a while before he went back to his cubicle.

'Thank you so much, Louise,' the nurse said to me before she carried on with the task she had been doing before she was interrupted.

'Don't worry about it. I don't mind being shouted at,' I told her.

13

Strangely Quiet

My night shift later that week was, dare I say it, quiet. I went in and saw Jim, one of the registrars, at the beginning of the shift.

'Is this your first night?' he asked.

'Yes,' I replied. 'You?'

'This is my third.'

'How have your nights been?' I continued.

'We had two shootings in last night,' he said.

Shootings have almost become a thing of the past and now we see more knife crime instead. To have two shootings in one night was unheard of. Jim told me that, fortunately, both turned out fine.

I sat down at the computer to see if anyone needed treatment. No one did and so I waited forty-five minutes for my first patient. I was so desperate for work that I went round asking everyone if they wanted help with anything or if any patients needed to go to the toilet. The answer was always no so I sat down again and waited. I sent a few messages to some of my friends who had just given birth because

I knew they'd be up feeding babies, 'I'm on a night shift. If you feel lonely, send me a message.'

Finally, a name appeared on the screen. I beat my doctor colleague to put my name beside it, indicating that I would be in charge of the patient's care. I read the brief description of what was wrong and discovered that this patient had been found collapsed on the street. I walked to his cubicle only to find no one there. I looked around. He had absconded. This was not a strong start to the shift. He must have made a quick exit because I hadn't wasted any time in making my way to see him.

The night went on and patients came trickling through, very slowly. There were various people who had taken overdoses, patients with chest pain and one woman had been sent in by the GP and was now hallucinating.

'I'm seeing people who I know aren't here,' she told me. 'One is standing behind you in the corner, just watching.'

Hallucinations can be linked to any number of medical problems. This woman needed to be admitted anyway for the issue she had originally presented with. She had come in feeling lethargic and confused and had low blood sodium, which could have been a cause of the hallucinations. Now it was a case for the medics on the ward to sort out.

Sometimes patients who hallucinate are so convinced that what they're seeing is real that they will grab thin air and swat away imaginary objects. They are very difficult for me to treat and there is no point in telling them that there's nothing there because they won't believe me. They're so perturbed that I also get scared but this patient was rational, thankfully.

Another lull followed. The department was already sparkling clean so there was nothing for me to tidy up. Instead, I passed the time chatting to my colleagues and was surprised by some of the things I learnt about them. Usually no one has time to breathe, let alone strike up a conversation that isn't patient-related, so this was a rare opportunity to delve into the lives of people I spend an inordinate amount of time with, yet knew little about.

A lot of people who work in healthcare have followed the traditional path into the profession. They've gone to university, done training and got a job. There are others, however, who have led a completely different life before starting to work in healthcare settings. In my department, we've got a nurse who used to be an engineer, a few doctors who are also Olympic athletes, a builder-turned-nurse, former lawyers and military personnel, and one healthcare assistant who is a personal bodyguard for celebrities in his spare time.

Our hospital workforce has diversity in all its forms under one roof. We've got managers and consultants at the top of their game earning hundreds of thousands of pounds a year alongside cleaners and porters on much less. We've got staff members from all around the world and from every socio-economic background.

It hadn't escaped us that most of the pictures of healthcare professionals who had died were those of people from a black and minority ethnic background. The trust had sent out messages asking anyone with worries to seek support from them. Some of my consultants had had to shield at home because coming into hospital was too risky for them.

The Black Lives Matter protests, brought about by a police officer killing George Floyd on 25 May in Minneapolis, were at the forefront of people's minds. There have been reports published that show the higher you go up the ranks in the health service, the number of BME staff decreases.

I'm not in a position to make a change on a big scale, but I would like to be one day. The NHS needs to push for more gender and racial equality otherwise it's shooting itself in the foot.

As my colleagues and I continued chatting, one nurse announced that she was leaving the NHS to be a fire fighter. I was surprised and sad because she had been such a fantastic colleague and nurse. I couldn't help but feel it was a loss for our hospital because she was one of the nicest, kindest and most empathetic people I had ever met. She was amazing.

I was also happy, however. It's so important to follow what you want to do. If nursing isn't for you, that's fine. There's no point in sticking with it. I think there are a lot of people working in the healthcare profession who probably shouldn't be. I've experienced as a patient nurses who have been really short tempered and who seem to have lost their compassion. When it gets to that point and you stop caring, you need to leave, but sometimes people just carry on because they don't have enough self-awareness.

All this made me think again how long it would be before I hung up my stethoscope. A&E definitely had a shelf life and I've always said it's a young person's game. There are older people who have stuck it out for years, but the majority are young. Typically, people come, get up-skilled quickly and then move on to somewhere with a slower pace of life. A&E is fast-paced and it's exhausting. I can maintain the lifestyle with shift work and working nights at the moment, but I can't see myself in this role for much longer than ten more years. I am thinking about having children, and trying to juggle that alongside shift work would be difficult, particularly because I have no family in the area. There's also the constant lure of a complete lifestyle change and I often dream of becoming a dog-walker or running a food van and going round festivals. I'd like to have time to expand on some of my hobbies and think about opening up my own cafe or exploring my creative side. The idea of not having to make life-and-death decisions under immense pressure is appealing.

The conversation then moved on to some of the horror stories from older members of staff who talked about how different hospitals were years ago. I thought back to what I'd seen and heard over my career. We've had patients in the hospital who have woken up in a delirious state and jumped out of windows to their death. A colleague found a nurse who had killed herself in one of the toilets on a night shift. I'd come in to work the next day and, even though no one knew her in A&E, the mood was black.

In the trust where I trained as a student nurse, there were always ghost stories. On one of my placements patients would often report seeing a boy in striped pyjamas. They'd also see a little girl stood by the window. In one of the side rooms, patients would recount being pushed down into the bed by an old lady. I didn't want to believe them and thought it might be some kind of sleep paralysis until one of the nurses went in for a nap on a night shift and it happened to her. Patients would scream until the nurses came in and at that point, it would stop. I was terrified and couldn't wait to finish that placement. I used to walk down the corridors with my back against the wall so I could see all around me. Whenever a patient buzzed in the middle of the night, I'd be so scared to attend them in case they told me they'd just seen a ghost.

I bet there are hundreds of similar stories in every hospital all over the world. I only know of one in my current hospital because I don't dare ask. There is one ward that is a twenty-minute walk away from A&E. In the corridors, they have lights that switch off to save energy and then come on when they detect movement. As you near the ward there is a circular mirror to help you see what's around the corner so you don't crash. Some of my colleagues have seen a white figure walking across the mirror but when they turned the corner, there was no one there. I've not experienced it myself though!

Our collective trip down memory lane came to an end when a new patient finally arrived and everyone dispersed. The computer said that this woman had smoked some marijuana and didn't feel well. I went in to see her and she was fast asleep, snoring. A collection of drool had pooled in the right corner of her mouth and was starting to roll down her chin. I woke her up and she looked disgusted with me.

'I'm so sorry to wake you,' I said.

'I'm hungry,' she replied.

I went off to find some food and returned with a sandwich. She gobbled it down.

'Oh, I feel so much better,' she said. 'I think I can go home now.'

I have had extensive medical training and none of it was needed for this patient. It had taken a sandwich to fix her. We get these cases from time to time. People come in drunk or high and sometimes sitting them up and giving them a coffee and something to eat works a treat. I discharged her and it wasn't long after that it was time to go home. It had been an odd night shift.

The next time I was in was over the weekend. My shift blurred into an amalgamation of patients who had attempted suicide and those who were victims of domestic violence. We were now in mid-June and the influx of domestic abuse survivors was getting worse as restrictions had eased. They were coming to A&E because, in some cases, they felt there was nowhere else to go even though services were still running. Not everyone knew what was available or how to get in touch with the right people. A&E is always open and the first place many people think of. I'd read that calls to the UK's national domestic helpline had reportedly risen by 66 per cent during lockdown and visits to its website increased by 950 per cent. Demand for beds in refuges had rocketed. Spaces were usually found but sometimes, we had to admit people overnight until one became available.

One woman had been beaten with a cricket bat and in other cases women's partners had tried to strangle and drown them as well as the kicking, hitting and punching. Two patients came in who were suicidal after months of verbal abuse and being told they were worthless. There were no refuge beds available because everything grinds to a halt over the weekend so they were all admitted into hospital and stayed until Monday. Many community services are also shut on Saturdays and Sundays with the majority of staff working Monday to Friday, 9 a.m. till 5 p.m., so it's hard to discharge patients if they need additional help. For that reason, the emergency department is usually at its busiest on a Sunday and Monday because there has been no movement from the hospital to other services.

The mental health side of things on that shift really got me thinking. Some patients had been brought in after sending pictures of empty pill packets or apologetic messages to friends who had then called an ambulance. I'd seen a few of them so many times before. The only thing I could do in A&E was to monitor their physical health, but their actions were clearly a cry for help and they needed to be listened to and validated.

This contrasted to other people I'd seen throughout my career who were absolutely determined to end their life. Those attempts were incredibly violent and no one else was aware of what they had been planning. I was reminded of the teenage boy who had gone to school in the morning as normal and come home at lunch to end his life. It was only by chance that his mother, who had dropped by to pick something up that she had forgotten in her rush to go to work in the morning, found him collapsed in his bedroom. I was a junior nurse at the time and I can still remember his face. He didn't make it. His mother was devastated and felt like she was responsible. She hadn't realized he was struggling.

'How did I not know this was happening?' she asked one of my senior colleagues when they broke the news to her.

Another woman had come in during lockdown saying she was finding things difficult, but was deemed fit to be discharged. The next day she was reported missing and those of us in the department had a sneaking suspicion that she had ended her life. Some days later her body was found in the canal. She had always intended to kill herself and did not want to be saved. The news rocked us. I was so glad I wasn't a specialist mental health professional. I do not envy them at all. Deciding whether to admit or discharge a patient on mental health grounds is the scariest type of responsibility in my view. So many patients will tell you, 'If you let me go, I'm going to kill myself.' Others are so withdrawn that they won't say anything. Trying to work out whether they will take action and the level of risk is astoundingly difficult.

At this point, the hospital's mental health services had started more face-to-face work but for a period they had to do the majority of their assessments over the phone. So much of making a decision is based on seeing the person in front of you, looking at their body language, seeing how well they are dressed, or whether they are underweight or overweight.

There was still a high number of mental health patients on my next shift. Some had turned up voluntarily, others were under section. The mental health team told me that if particular individuals tried to leave, then it was my responsibility to enforce a section. I felt completely out of my depth with all the different sections and what each one meant. There are so many and they tell you what level of restraint you can enforce and for how long. Everything is enshrined in law because depriving someone of their freedom is serious and you have to make sure you are doing the right thing. I hoped against hope that nobody would kick up a fuss.

Often, I find I can talk patients down when they are in crisis in the department, but sometimes we have to physically and chemically restrain them. There are guidelines and there is always someone very senior involved because, understandably, there's a great deal of controversy around restraining patients and it needs to be done safely, otherwise people can die. It once took eight members of staff, myself included, to restrain one patient. He was off his face on drugs and was phenomenally strong. We had one person holding each lower leg, thigh, arm and his shoulders, and one to insert a cannula to mildly sedate him. It was dangerous, sweaty, hard work and we were doing it for the safety of the patient. He had no capacity to make decisions for himself and we were concerned that if he was left unsedated, he would fling himself off the trolley, hit his head or break his neck and kill himself in the process. That would come back on us as negligence because he was under our care.

It got to the end of my shift and all my patients with mental health problems had remained calm. I breathed a sigh of relief and went home to read up on all the sections that existed and their implications.

After all that reading, I still didn't feel confident

that I knew everything there was to know, so I was thankful I was working in minors the next day. There was little to no likelihood that I would be seeing any suicidal patients there. Nevertheless, it was a frustrating shift because I spent most of it on the phone to various specialities. We'd had several weeks at the height of the virus, where referring patients to other areas of the hospital was a dream because everyone was so obliging. That golden period had now ended. Theoretically, if we call a speciality from A&E, they are meant to take the patient. If they then think we've got it wrong, it's up to them to transfer that patient to the correct speciality. That day, it wasn't working like that.

'I've got a patient who needs to be with you in the frailty department,' I started. 'Her respiratory rate is a little low, but . . .'

'She needs to go to Respiratory,' a voice barked back.

I rang Respiratory.

'Hello, I've got a patient here for you. Frailty won't take her because she's got breathing problems.'

'OK, what else?'

'She's got a fractured pelvis but I'll tell you now that there's nothing that needs to be done with it, she'll just need painkillers and for it to be mobilized.'

'Oh no, you need to check with Orthopaedics. Can you phone Orthopaedics to confirm, please? We can't take her otherwise.'

I phoned Orthopaedics.

'Yes, nothing to be done with that fractured pelvis. She's fine to go to Respiratory.'

I rang Respiratory again.

'Hello, it's me with the patient who needs to come up to you. Orthopaedics are happy that they don't need to see her.'

I felt like some kind of negotiator and that I was wasting time flipping between various hospital departments. It was annoying that this situation had suddenly got better for the peak of the pandemic before taking a turn for the worse. Perhaps they were stressed about the vast workload coming their way as more NHS services that had been put on hold resumed and were faced with huge backlogs.

Another department I called with alarming frequency that day was Urology. I was sure that they were fed up with me and I could imagine their hearts sinking when they heard it was A&E on the phone as it meant more work on top of their already crammed schedule. I called multiple times about a patient who couldn't pee, another one who was pissing blood, someone who had a strange kidney disease which I'd probably never see or hear of again in my career, and last but not least, a man who had inserted three safety pins up his urethra.

'He's done what?' said the urology registrar, perking up after obviously switching off when he first heard my voice.

Up until I saw this man, my day had mostly been filled with run-of-the-mill procedures. Almost everyone

I had seen had complained of chest pain or that they didn't feel very well. I had walked into this cubicle and started off with my customary greeting, 'Hiya, my name's Louise. What's brought you into A&E today?'

'I've shoved some safety pins up my penis,' came the reply.

'Oh yes? OK then, I'm just going to ask you some questions to enable me to know how to treat you.'

I followed up with a number of queries around when he'd done this and why. Did he have any other problems? Was he suffering from tummy pain, could he wee, did his urine look normal? Was it painful when he went to the toilet?

'I did it as a form of release,' he told me after answering everything else. 'I've got a lot of emotional pain that haunts me and doing things like this sometimes help with taking it away.'

I ordered an X-ray of his pelvis, which confirmed that there were indeed three safety pins lodged inside his body and sent him straight up to be treated by Urology.

Some people do things like this for sexual pleasure. I'm not sure what pleasure is derived from it, as we didn't cover that in my training, but I guess it's some kind of fetish, or they get a thrill from experiencing pain. Shoving objects up the urethra can cause a lot of damage. First of all, there's a lot of blood and if you were to put a camera up there, you'd see tearings in the wall. It can also cause infections and all sorts of structural problems.

I looked up my next patient and saw at the same time that the isolation units had been empty for at least an hour. That was the first time that had happened when I'd been on shift. Murmurs of 'Oh, that's good' went round the department. Certainly the number of Covid-19 cases and deaths had drastically tailed off over the past month but I wasn't sure if this was a true reflection of whether we were over the worst of it or whether there was more to come. One thing we all knew was that the pandemic had not ended, and it wasn't long before the two isolation units we still had open were brimming with patients again.

I also saw one of our regulars for the third time that week, and the number of patients walking into A&E with complaints that could have been dealt with by the GP was rapidly increasing and approaching pre-lockdown levels. In the midst of lockdown, we'd have no more than ten people in minors but this had increased to thirty in there at the same time.

A lot of people omitted information when they were booked in at reception so I ended up seeing a man with ankle pain that had been going on for months. This was not an accident, or an emergency.

'You need to go and see your GP,' I told him, at which point he erupted in anger.

'I can't see my GP because they're only doing appointments over the phone!'

I was reminded of a time when a man came in complaining that his antibiotics weren't working.

'How long have you been taking them?' I asked.

'I started them a few hours ago,' he replied.

It was clear that the general public continued to think that we were over the worst of the pandemic. I could understand why; numbers of daily deaths were decreasing, restrictions were easing and perhaps it wasn't realistic to expect people to live on high alert for months on end. The situation in A&E was well along the path to returning to the way it was before coronavirus hit.

It was Ed's birthday and we celebrated it by going on another walk with the dogs to a local beauty spot. In the evening we ordered pizza and had some drinks down by the river. Luckily the weather was pleasant and we played a board game. Ed and I are big fans of board games. We have amassed more than twenty over the years and we're always on the lookout for new ones.

We took a taxi that night and I was surprised when the driver told me not to bother putting on my face mask. He wasn't wearing one. I decided to wear mine anyway. I couldn't help feeling confused by how much the guidance had changed over the trajectory of the pandemic; previously people had dismissed face masks, now they were mandatory on public transport. It reminded me of the constantly changing PPE requirements at the beginning of the crisis.

Back at work and it was a bog-standard day in A&E – a couple of heart attacks and loads of recreational drug use. I guessed people had more time on their hands now that many were on furlough or had lost their jobs and so passed the day by dabbling in a whole range of mind-altering substances, including amphetamines, spice, cocaine, pain medication, cannabis and more. Some had come in by ambulance after a passer-by had seen them collapsed in a street or an alley, while others had brought themselves in because they were worried about chest pain or palpitations.

We can't do much for people in situations like these. Unless someone has taken opiates, we don't tend to prescribe an antidote because that can lead to more problems like seizures, so we monitor them until their high fades.

There is a database we use that tells us how long to monitor a patient and what kind of effects each drug has. Does it cause an irregular heartbeat or fits or can it lead to cardiac arrest? It lists what to prescribe in each situation in case of low blood pressure or a high heart rate. In particular cases, people may get a high temperature of 40 degrees which is really dangerous and so we put ice packs in their arm pits and groin. Sometimes the sedation effects of a drug can cause people to lose the ability to maintain their airway and then we have to intubate them. One person's afternoon of fun can turn out to be hellish.

We get a lot of patients coming through the doors who take heroin. If they've taken too much, we give them a drug which reverses the effects of it. The patient will be conked out in front of you, you'll give them the drug and within seconds they'll sit bolt upright. I always take five steps back after I've administered it because people can go manic and start fighting you if you're too close. Sometimes they'll be angry and accuse me of ruining their trip.

I always struggle to understand people when they say what they've taken because I had a sheltered upbringing and the terminology and vocabulary is vast. There are so many different words for the various drugs and the amount that's taken.

One man came in and said he'd taken blind squid.

'I don't know what that is,' I replied.

'Cat valium?'

'Sorry?'

'Super acid?'

'What?'

'Vitamin K?'

'Huh?'

'Ketamine?'

'Ah, OK, why didn't you say that in the first place? How much did you take?'

'Fifty pounds' worth.'

'Is that a lot?'

I ask people to explain all the time and they're very obliging and don't mind. There's also a website which lists loads of slang terms which is useful. Recently, when I asked how much they'd taken, patients would use the term 'keys' which completely baffled me. Did they put the drug on a key? How big was the key? How many grooves had it got? Or was 'key' some kind of slang for a volume or measurement?

Drugs can make people really aggressive and hyper alert or they can lead to someone being completely out of it. A lot of people tell me I'm beautiful which is lovely, until I realize it's probably the drugs talking.

Next up was a woman who had come in complaining of chest pain. I performed an ECG which looked fine but I was still waiting for the results of her blood tests, one of which would indicate whether she had had a heart attack. She didn't want to wait and so walked off while I was attending to someone else.

A while later her blood test came back and showed that she had indeed suffered a heart attack. I found her number on her patient records and called it. She answered.

'Heyyyyyy, it's Louise from A&E.'

'Oh. Er, hi.'

'How are you doing? Still got a bit of chest pain?'

'Yes, actually. It does hurt a bit.'

'Well, that makes sense, your blood test shows you've probably had a heart attack. Would you like to come back?'

'Oh. Er, OK, if I must.'

Four hours later she strolled back in to the department with a considerably pinker face than before. She had obviously been sitting out in the sun enjoying a few alcoholic drinks. We sent her straight to the cardio ward for treatment.

She was in contrast to my other patient that day with a heart attack who was so panicked it was hard to tell whether her chest pain was due to cardiac damage or overwhelming anxiety.

The rest of the day was taken up with people who were struggling with the heat. It was sweltering outside and there wasn't a cloud in the sky. I saw patients who had collapsed while out shopping, or felt bad after spending all day in the sun after a heavy drinking session the night before. The number of acute kidney injuries, brought about by dehydration, stacked up as time marched on.

I got home after my shift and sat down to watch the news. It was 25 June, a hot day, and there were images of Bournemouth beach crammed with people. The pictures were everywhere and a major incident had been declared. I was furious and so were my colleagues. One wrote on a work Facebook group that he was raging. He and his wife had worked opposite rotas in high-risk areas of the NHS with children at home and it was galling to see people flout all the guidance because the sun was out.

I know what a major incident feels like because I've worked through them in the hospital. Hospitals would be seeing an influx of drunk or sunburnt patients, both problems self-inflicted, and adding pressure to already overburdened services.

The next day, Ed and I were listening to the radio in the car when a caller rang in and blamed the government for the whole fiasco. This just made me angrier. I could certainly see that the government's messaging around guidelines wasn't clear at all, and of course I was eagerly awaiting the results of an inquiry into what had gone wrong, but it wasn't their fault that loads of people had all gone to the same beach at the same time.

At this point the death toll each day in the UK was still surpassing 100 and there were thousands of new cases. Worldwide, the virus was running rampant through the US, India and Brazil. Cities in China had also already locked down again after outbreaks were discovered.

We were also gearing up for the weekend of 4 July in A&E. Pubs were due to open again and extra shifts were being advertised. Super Saturday, as it was labelled, was going to be utter carnage. I'd noticed in the city centre that people were all over the place and not sticking to the one-way system. I didn't dare imagine what would happen when they'd had a few drinks.

14

Road Traffic Accidents

Back in A&E, we were all starting to feel the pressure of having only two isolation units open. The third had by this point been returned to its former glory as part of minors. It was imperative that we did not exceed capacity in isolation as there was nowhere else to put Covid patients; they'd have to stay on the ambulance until there was room. If that happened, that vehicle would be out of action and unable to get back on the road and pick up other people who might be in danger. All of us working in the isolation units knew we had to act and make decisions quickly, especially when both were full, which was happening quite a lot. I knew the overall number of coronavirus cases was dropping – our daily emails from the trust were now appearing in my inbox only three times a week. When coronavirus was at its peak, we'd have hundreds of confirmed and suspected cases and every day for weeks the numbers didn't change. Now it was down to just below 100 confirmed and suspected combined.

I didn't think many of my patients on one of my

night shifts in isolation had Covid-19. Anyone who was short of breath or had chest pain was a possibility though and had to come via the isolation unit unless it was glaringly obvious that their symptoms were attributable to something else. Once they were in the unit, we would take a closer look at them and move them on, if appropriate. While shortness of breath was a definite marker of coronavirus, it was also a factor in a load of other medical conditions.

It got to 6 a.m. and there was a rush of patients. Older people had got out of bed and collapsed on the floor sustaining head injuries, hip and rib fractures, or collapsed lungs. Others had gone to bed feeling ill but had hoped they would feel better in the morning. When they woke up and realized they had deteriorated, it wasn't long before they were in with us.

Outside of the isolation unit that night, the cold resus had been busy dealing with road traffic collisions, or RTCs for short. When I had a chance to pause for a moment to think, I realized we hadn't had anywhere near as many of these for a long time during lockdown. Now numbers of crashes were getting back to normal. There were two in that night. One was a drunk driver who crashed into a tree and hadn't been wearing a seatbelt. He died shortly after arriving. The other was a woman in her thirties who had recently got married and had a baby at home. She came in fully alert but suddenly tanked and then arrested. In a last-ditch attempt to save her life, the team cut open her chest to look for where blood was escaping and to clamp the aorta to stop it supplying the lower limbs and focus on the vital organs. It's a brutal procedure and only done when absolutely necessary. Unfortunately, she didn't make it. The other driver involved in the crash hadn't come into the department. I guessed that they had escaped without injuries because they were in a much larger vehicle.

When I was a more junior nurse, I'd often be in charge of the resus department and RTCs were a frequent occurrence. If it was a bit icy or if it had been raining overnight, it would get to 7 a.m. and the red phone was guaranteed to go off with news that someone would be turning up who had usually skidded in a vehicle. I'd be due to finish in an hour and on my last legs and would have to rally the whole team and get a bay ready to receive a trauma patient and make sure we had all the right equipment.

Apart from that we also see a lot of hit and runs and people driving with too many others in the back. It's gut-wrenching when we have victims of a crash where five or six people have crammed into a car with only four seat belts. All too often the person sat in the middle of the back seat has shot through the windscreen and died. It's usually a group of eighteen-year-olds and the driver has recently passed their test and got their licence. I can only imagine the overwhelming guilt and regret the driver must be left with for the rest of their life.

It doesn't escape me that one day it could be someone

I know that comes in to resus. I try not to think about all the victims of car crashes I see outside of work because that is no way to live. I sometimes worry about Ed when he cycles or drives, though, because he gets so tired. He's come off his bike two or three times before and once he even ended up in A&E. The first I found out was when I rang him from home where I was waiting for him to get back so we could eat supper together. He answered and I asked, 'Where are you? I'm hungry.'

'I'm at work.'

'Why are you still there?'

'No, I'm at your work.'

My stomach plummeted.

'What the hell has happened?'

'I'm OK. I was hit by a car coming out of a junction. I went over the bonnet and landed on the road. I'm badly bruised and have strained some muscles but I'll live.'

After I'd heard about the patients that had been involved in road traffic collisions and had come into cold resus, I went to see if my colleague needed any help with his patient who was perilously close to cardiac arrest. The man's breathing was terrible and he looked awful. The doctor dealing with him was hugely busy so I offered to phone the family. His wife picked up.

'Hello, my name's Louise and I'm calling from A&E. Your husband is incredibly unwell and I think you should come down.'

'But I thought visitors weren't allowed into the hospital?' she said.

'I think we can make an exception in this case. Come down to be with your husband.'

'Oh God, OK I'll be there as soon as I can. You're sure it's OK for me to come in?'

'Yes. Ask for me when you get here. Just to add, you need to understand that you will be coming into a hospital that is caring for Covid patients. You'll need to wear PPE and there is a risk of contracting the virus.'

'I understand,' she replied.

'Is there someone who can bring you?' I asked. The last thing I wanted was for her to drive to the hospital in a panic and end up in a road traffic collision. We'd already had those two fatalities that evening.

'My son can bring me.'

When his wife arrived, the intensive care doctor came to talk to her and the patient was taken up to ICU. I finished my night shift not knowing how long he would survive, but I knew he was in the best place and I went home to try and sleep.

I had my weekly video call with my mum and sister the next day. Mum updated me on the goings-on in their village. There had been three non-coronavirus-related deaths and people had stood outside their front doors to watch the hearses go by. It reminded me of when we said farewell to my father. Seeing his coffin and then driving behind it was difficult. Some idiot managed to get in between the hearse and my mum's car at the exact wrong moment in a village which is completely out of the way and usually has very little traffic. I could see my sister's arms waving frantically, motioning for him to get out of the way. I was surprised she didn't reach across and beep the horn or get out and yell at him.

Apart from that, the day had been weirdly lovely and we were so overwhelmed by how many people turned up to the service of thanksgiving. My mum thought forty people would come and then about half that for drinks afterwards. There'd be enough room in our house for that. My sister wasn't so sure, so she rang the funeral director to get more service sheets printed off, and we decided last minute to hold the wake in the village hall.

A fair few of my father's friends couldn't make it because they lived so far away and were elderly themselves, but even so the church was packed. We were so touched by all these people who came to mourn my dad's passing, but also celebrate his life. Afterwards, the village hall was also busy. We had an open bar because Dad was always a great host and firmly believed that his guests shouldn't pay for anything. Our neighbour ran the bar that afternoon and said things picked up after my sister went and ordered a bottle of Prosecco to share with friends.

Back on our video chat and Mum told me about the local church service that was being held over a telephone conference line.

'Why isn't it done online?' I asked.

'This is rural North Yorkshire. I'm one of the youngest people who regularly attends our church and I'm seventy. Some people don't use the internet.'

'Oh, right.'

'It's largely fine but you can hear people breathing. Also, we've only just learned to not sing along to the hymns and listen instead. When people sing, it breaks up the lovely music.'

She's got this way of making the mundane and ordinary seem hilarious. I'll never forget her relaying various incidents, like somebody in the village spraying 'twat' in weedkiller on another person's lawn, or the time her and my dad had people round for drinks and a neighbour spilt red wine on the light beige carpet. She and my ex-military dad kept the house spotless. He was probably the bigger neat freak of the two and immediately went to get the carpet cleaner and got down on his knees and started scrubbing in front of everyone.

As the conversation was drawing to a close, my sister prompted my mum to talk about last night's supper. My sister had prepared her first meal since living there for months. They had eaten salmon with a potato salad and asparagus. Mum said the potatoes and asparagus were undercooked but that it was otherwise very good. They were alive and not suffering with diarrhoea and vomiting so my sister was pretty chuffed. She has had a tumultuous relationship with cooking over the years. Aged fifteen, she managed to fill the house with green smoke while making popcorn and she's been known to cook pizza with the polystyrene base still attached. Mostly, my mum tells her to keep away from the kitchen.

Not long after we finished talking, I went to work my second night shift in a row. There's an unwritten rule that when you work nights, it's compulsory to have a conversation around how many hours' sleep you managed to get. It never comes up on a day shift. That evening, my colleague told me she had slept for ten hours. TEN HOURS! I couldn't believe it because I had only managed to get a measly three and a half hours.

That night, I was in majors and it was another typical A&E sort of shift. Three overdoses, one heart attack, two suspected strokes, one renal stone and one deep vein thrombosis. To manage some of the horrors we go through in A&E, the team really pulls together and one coping mechanism is to make jokes about each other. People pick on me for the way I talk (they think I'm posh), they think I'm too nice, that I'm naive because I don't know anything about drugs, and that I get 'hangry'. If people don't know who I am but need to find me, they'll ask and my colleagues will point to me and label me 'the tall, pretty posh girl'. It's all good-humoured banter and I give as good as I get, or try to. I always think of witty comebacks too late.

I managed to do some teaching to some junior colleagues. I'm often struck by imposter syndrome and waiting to be told that I'm not good enough to do the job of an ACP. Sometimes, it's difficult to take a step back and see how far I've come. In that moment when I managed to answer some of the questions thrown at me, I realized that I could do the job. It was a small confidence boost.

After that I went to see a woman who had taken a cocktail of drugs and washed them down with a bottle of vodka. As I was doing my assessment, I asked if there was any chance she could be pregnant.

'Definitely not,' came the answer.

'OK, and when was your last period?'

'Hmm, not sure. Maybe three weeks ago? I don't really keep track.'

I went to check her medical records and, lo and behold, they showed that she had had an ultrasound two weeks previously and that she was expecting a baby. I went back to her.

'Your medical records state that you had an ultra-sound a couple of weeks ago and that you are definitely pregnant.'

She looked guilty. 'Oh, er, it must have slipped my mind.'

'Right, well, you know drinking this amount of alcohol and taking these substances puts you and your unborn baby's health at serious risk?'

At that point, she broke down in tears.

'I just want it to go! I don't want to have it. I can't look after myself let alone another human being and the father has left me. I don't know what to do and I've had enough!'

I was annoyed that she'd lied to me but it wasn't

the first, and it wouldn't be the last, time that had happened. I also felt desperately sad that she was in this situation and appeared to be alone. She had to stay the night in hospital under observation so I rang the ward and the safeguarding team, who would hopefully be able to help her more than I could.

My final patient of the night hadn't left his house in many years. He was only in A&E because his medical problem was so bad that he couldn't survive on his own at home. His skin was dry and had a brown tinge to it. His clothes were heavily soiled in urine and faeces. When I took off his socks, dry skin was blown up into the air creating what I can only describe as a snow storm. I held my breath and then inhaled as gently as I could, just in case some of the dead skin flakes had fallen behind my mask.

His nails were long and stained brown by the countless cigarettes he smoked. I was desperate to give this man a good long soak in the bath. I'd have to make do with changing him into a hospital gown and giving him a wet wipe wash. Just with that he already looked a million times better.

As I was tending to him I began trying to find out how he had got himself into this situation.

'How has it been at home? Have you been managing?'

'Oh yes, apart from these last few days I've been fine,' he replied. 'I don't like going out so I just stay at home. I don't have any friends or family so there's no reason to leave the house.'

'Who's been doing your shopping?'

'One of the people down the road does it and drops it off outside my door.'

'And who does your cooking and cleaning?'

'I do the bare minimum. I've never really enjoyed housework and it's only me living there.'

'Are you able to get to the shower? Do you have a bath?'

'I've got arthritis now so it's a bit of a challenge,' he admitted.

'Do you think you might need some help?'

'Oh, I don't know. I don't think so. I wouldn't want to trouble anyone,' he replied.

I wondered how many more people were living in similar situations and lying undiscovered at home. We see recluses and cases of neglect quite often in A&E; they're almost always older people who have been ravaged by loneliness. I remember one woman who hadn't stepped outside her front door in fifteen years. Her nephew did anything she needed so she didn't have to leave home. When she finally turned up at hospital, cancer had eaten half her face down to her eyeballs.

Lockdown would have made it far easier for people to be forgotten, and it would have dragged others who were just managing down into a whirlpool of despair. How many individuals without many friends or family had been forced to stay inside and had now sunk further into a vicious quicksand of loneliness and boredom? As people continued to decline physically and mentally,

I thought we would probably see the after-effects in A&E over the next weeks and months.

My patient needed to be admitted for his medical problems. At least that gave us some time to refer him to services and charities that might be able to help and to sort out a care package for him when he returned home.

I had the following day off but I felt time was running away with me. I had dog walks to do, I was meeting a couple of friends in town and had to get the bus there, and I had a load of ironing and other chores to do at home. I also had book club in the evening and hadn't finished reading that fortnight's title. What's more, my dissertation, the last task I had to complete before gaining my MSc in advanced clinical practice, was hanging over me and wasn't going to write itself.

I was also still trying to make up around nine hours' sleep deficit from when I was working nights. I woke up and left at 9.45 a.m. to get the bus into town but stood at the stop for ages, waiting. When I got into town, one of my friends was an hour late in arriving so I didn't get back to the house till 3 p.m. I was relieved when some of the book club members revealed they also had not finished the latest book. I was over halfway through but could not have told you the names of the main characters or the storyline, because it was so bad. The person leading it announced that we wouldn't have a chat about it that evening which was a relief but I knew I'd still have to finish the blasted thing. The thought of switching on my Kindle and seeing a book 57 per cent completed was too much to bear. I hate not finishing things. Before I could completely relax, the group were asking me for recommendations for the next read. I panicked and left my sister a stricken voice note.

'Oh my god, I'm panicking. The book club are asking me for a book suggestion because I haven't made one yet. I need to look good so can you please suggest an up-and-coming – or whatever – really good book for us to read pronto? Thanks. Bye.'

My sister messaged back: 'OMG don't panic me like that.' This year had also been tough for her and she'd got used to people revealing awful things both in her personal and professional life as a journalist. She sent me a load of suggestions which I fed into the group chat. My sister may have a ridiculous, stroppy and hilarious side to her, but she also reads a lot, is opinionated and is usually abreast of what's coming out, what's been hailed by critics, as well as various trends.

Back at work the next day I was in the isolation unit again. Just as we'd reduced our capacity and staffing levels for the hot side of A&E, it emerged that new hotspots were popping up in various areas around the country. Leicester was going to be the only city that didn't lift existing restrictions on businesses, including pubs, opening on 4 July because there had been a noticeable spike in cases there. It was starting to feel inevitable that we also might have a surge in cases again. Was the dreaded second wave that people had been talking about for months on its way? Not only that, but the upcoming weekend with all the pubs opening was making everyone nervous. Some news reports were predicting it would be like New Year's Eve. I've worked a few of them in my time and they can get messy.

It's always at about 10 p.m. that the trickle of ambulances bringing in drunk patients turns into a steady flow. Patients are either alone and have lost control of all their bodily functions or they come accompanied by a small group of friends. That wouldn't be happening with current restrictions on hospital visitors in place, though. Instead, the department would be carrying the extra workload created by intoxicated fun-seekers on top of everything else and all the possible Covid patients. People would still be ill, and accidents were almost guaranteed to happen.

The first patient of the day had been feeling short of breath for a week. Her chest X-ray revealed signs of Covid. I explained: 'It looks like you have pneumonia in both your lungs, which could mean you have the virus.'

She looked at me, shocked. 'But I haven't left the house in weeks!'

'Has anyone come to see you?'

'Yes, a few people. Family mostly. I can't really survive on my own at home without help.'

'It might have come from them,' I said gently. Here was another person who had fallen victim to this awful virus because she was vulnerable and her family had tried to help and care for her. She was reasonably well though and I wasn't too worried.

'I expect you'll be discharged in a day or so,' I reassured her before I said goodbye as she was transferred up to the ward.

As I turned around to get on with my next job, my consultant called me to help with a cardiac arrest that was imminent. She was wheeled in by the paramedics, who explained she had had a downtime of just under two hours, meaning that she had been in cardiac arrest for that length of time, needing CPR and not showing any sign of improvement. Her chances of survival were slim to nothing but her heart was in a shockable rhythm and so we kept trying. We got the defibrillator pads out and set them to charge. The jolt as the electricity charged through her body was a harsh and very visual reminder of what a violent procedure resuscitation is. Her arms were strapped in and hugging the Lucas machine as it continuously pumped away at her chest. We gave her three rounds of adrenalin and three shocks but her heart soon went into a non-shockable rhythm. She had been in cardiac arrest now for over two hours. We discussed what to do as a team and the decision was made to stop.

I barely had time to reflect and check in on the two student nurses who had just witnessed their first ever cardiac arrest before another patient was pushed through the doors. They looked a similar shade of grey to the patient we'd just tried to resuscitate. This day was turning out to be really stressful.

The ambulance crew who handed the patient over knew very little about him and he was too unwell to talk to me. He was short of breath and using every muscle he could in an effort to get oxygen into his lungs. His oxygen saturations were at 52 per cent, which is terrible. They should have been above 90 per cent. His chest sounded like a whistling train. Despite the racket of the chaos going on around me, the sound of his chest was deafening. His blood gases showed that he was in respiratory failure. He was not in a good way.

I prescribed a load of drugs to try to open up his airways and improve his breathing. While my nursing colleagues were busy making up the medicines, I did some detective work and tried to find out as much as I could about my patient. I looked back through his records to see if he had been to A&E before, or had any clinic letters. I couldn't find out anything. When the drugs were ready, we pumped them into him and waited.

After two hours of back-to-back nebulizers, steroids and magnesium, my patient was a new man. He could talk to me, even if it was only three words at a time. This was an amazing improvement. His blood gases were moving in the right direction and I felt like I'd achieved something massive. I, and my colleagues, had helped stop this man inching towards the point of no return.

Another patient in cardiac arrest came crashing through the doors and this time my colleague took charge. I was happy to hear later that the patient survived and had regained a pulse and a blood pressure, but only time would tell if she would ever recover enough to leave the hospital.

What a day. I got on my bike and on the ride home, a man wolf whistled at me. Pathetic. I ignored him and then later got annoyed at myself for not yelling a witty comeback that he would have heard as I rode past.

15

The Best and Worst of People

Back in majors, I was left on my own as the only clinician for a few hours while all available staff were sent to minors, which was heaving.

The department had changed again overnight. A second isolation unit had closed and been returned to its original state. We were left with just one unit with ten beds. The numbers of cold patients were far exceeding those with suspected Covid and we still had social-distancing measures to take into account so had to create more space to work in. We had still got patients with Covid fighting for their lives in intensive care and I was anxious about reducing our capacity to care for others with coronavirus. So far, more than 43,000 people had died deaths linked to Covid-19 in the UK. Daily deaths had fallen to below 100 on most days, but we were all painfully aware there might be a second wave.

Every hour I got a pop-up message on my computer screen reminding me of the anticipated increase in numbers this weekend as pubs were due to reopen.

They were asking any staff who were available to work extra shifts. I thought about it – the extra pay would be welcome after all – but I had a sixty-hour week ahead of me and needed some time to decompress and rest. My mental health had taken a battering over the past few weeks and my confidence was wavering.

I saw a patient who was in a state of diabetic emergency. She was slumped on the bed and fidgeting with clammy skin because she'd been sweating so much. Her glucose levels were so high that our machines were unable to read them and give us a result.

'I can't get a reading for your blood sugar levels,' I told her. 'They are astronomically high.'

'Hmm, I may have been a little over-indulgent during lockdown. I've got a bit of a thing for Terry's chocolate oranges,' she says. 'I've been having one every other day.'

While listening to her confessions about her secret eating, I reflected on my own bad habits. I had certainly gained a few kilos since lockdown had started.

'Erm, I've also been baking cakes every day and having them for pudding with a dollop of cream on top. But they are homemade.'

'Right. I'm sure they have less preservatives than shop-bought ones, but they'll still be full of butter and sugar. You need to try and cut down on the sweet stuff. Can you book an appointment with your diabetic nurse specialist to discuss what alterations you can make to your diet?'

'Yes. I know it all already. I think it's just because I've had nothing much else to do and have been comfort eating. I tend to do that when I'm anxious.'

While she had been over-indulging during lockdown, I was suspicious that there might be another reason why her sugars and other results were so deranged. When the lab phoned through with her glucose result, it confirmed which type of diabetic emergency she was in. She was transferred to resus where she could be more closely monitored while an insulin infusion was set up. She needed one-to-one care with regular blood sugar checks to monitor her glucose levels and make sure she didn't go into a hypoglycaemic coma.

The rest of my shift was taken up with treating women who had suffered domestic abuse. One had tried to take her own life because she'd tried to escape but been caught every time. She couldn't take any more. She told me: 'At least if I'm dead, he can't hurt me. He's got weapons at home and he inflicts so much pain on me. Please, he can't see me here.'

She had started to panic and so I tried to reassure her. 'One good thing in this case about the pandemic is that we're not letting any visitors in. They're not allowed. You're safe in here.'

The drugs she had taken in an attempt to end her life were no doubt exacerbating her fears and anxiety. They were in her system and there was little else I could do. She needed monitoring, but more importantly, she needed to be kept safe. As she was taken up to the ward I phoned the police to report the weapons and carried out a safeguarding referral so the team would see her as soon as possible.

The other woman I saw had left her abusive partner and been placed in a temporary safe house where he couldn't find her. She'd recently left and was just starting out in her life without him when he found her and beat her almost to death. She had multiple rib fractures, a lung contusion and a bleed on the brain. I couldn't imagine what she had endured to get into this state or how he could have kept hitting her to inflict all these injuries. It was also gut-wrenching that she had built up the courage to leave him and was just starting to get on with her life when he crashed back into it and destroyed all the progress she had made. She was admitted for further treatment and I hoped that once she got out, she would have the strength to carry on living and find happiness away from abusive men.

That shift had taken it out of me. I felt physically and emotionally battered after a tough couple of weeks and headed straight home. I was so thankful I wasn't working over the upcoming weekend, with the 4 July easing of a load of restrictions in England. I couldn't believe that pubs were opening while people in hospital still couldn't have visitors unless they were at death's door, and even then only one person was allowed in. It somehow didn't seem fair. I spared a thought for my colleagues who were on duty and I wondered what the future now held for us in A&E.

One thing was certain, we had a long struggle in front of us. The numbers of people attending were on the rise and I shuddered with dread at the thought of how we would cope when winter came around. But then, I thought again, and marvelled at how we in the NHS had nimbly and effectively managed the tsunami of coronavirus patients that had threatened to drown us and destroy everything in its way. We were a hair's breadth away from being overwhelmed but we'd coped and delivered outstanding care at every turn while everything around us was in a state of chaotic flux. I knew we would continue to weather any storm together, and in that respect I wasn't alone. We would face whatever was to come together.

I also thought of the bravery I'd seen from my patients who were going through horrors in circumstances that most people couldn't have imagined as little as six months previously. The vast majority were brave, kind, wise and charming people. I thought of the older generations who had lived through wars and died without the love and reassurance of their families. I had been there as they inched closer to death's embrace or even as they had slipped away while I, a stranger, whose face was covered by a mask stripping me of most of my humanity, looked on and held their hand. I was humbled by their dignity and courage.

I also remembered the people who had clung on and been saved against all the odds and wondered what they were doing now. Had they fully recovered? Had their outlook changed after such an experience and what were they doing with their lives?

As for me, all year I'd felt as if I were in the process of doing a somersault underwater and had lost which way was up to the surface. My own life had been rocked by my father's death and then working through what I hoped would be this once-in-a-lifetime health crisis. For the first time, I'd skirted around and occasionally plunged into a black hole of poor mental health. I knew I wasn't the only one and wondered what toll this would take on the NHS workforce. I felt pulled in all directions at work but also in my personal life. I couldn't be there as much as I wanted for my grieving mother.

I looked back at the wild rollercoaster ride that 2020 had been so far and laughed at some of the more bizarre elements of it. Had supermarket shelves across the country really been stripped of all toilet roll? I still couldn't get my head round that. Had people really said, 'It's only a flu, why all the fuss?' Had the president of the US actually suggested injecting bleach as a cure for Covid-19?

I'd seen how this pandemic had brought out the best and worst in people and it had revealed their true nature with blistering clarity. There had been confirmations of what I thought I knew, but also surprises. I'd been moved to the core by people's outward celebrations of the NHS and their gratitude. I finally felt seen, and to have my job recognized in such a way was life-affirming. Although the weekly clapping had stopped, people still felt passionate about what an amazing institution the health service was. I hoped that line of thought would stick around because it had buoyed me and my colleagues when we really needed it.

I was proud of my contribution. I've said before that I don't have a faith, but some small part of me wondered if there was some higher presence guiding me through life. I couldn't begin to formulate in my mind why things happened the way they did but I started to feel like my role caring for others at their greatest moment of need was a calling and one of my true purposes in life. Had I been put on this earth to be there with people at their lowest ebb and to help them up and out of one of the worst times in their lives? For me there was no greater privilege, even if it was scary, overwhelming and frustrating all at the same time.

The loss of hundreds of health workers to coronavirus was devastating. A public inquiry was yet to happen but I wondered how many people had been lost because of systemic failings. Seeing colleagues around the country work in dangerous circumstances without the adequate protection had sent shudders down my spine.

I thought about all those people whose lives had been punched by grief. I had a feeling the fallout of people not being able to grieve as normal was yet to come. I also pondered those whose lives had been changed irrevocably during lockdown. People had struggled with loneliness and mental health problems before restrictions hit. How had they fared? We were in recession and the economic consequences of the pandemic meant that more families had been plunged into poverty. With that would come a whole host of health issues. I knew that we in the NHS would be picking up the pieces for months to come and it would be in A&E where we saw the sharp end of the destruction wrought on people's lives.

Throughout it all, individuals' generosity and selflessness had been incredible. Communities had rallied to look after the needy. Those of us working in A&E had received hot meals, countless offers and discounts as well as gift bags with freebies. People had sewed scrubs for us. I'd never forget the thank you cards I was sent, or the volunteers who had done all manner of tasks to help out.

Alongside that though ran a stream of selfishness. I guessed this pandemic had given people time to re-evaluate their lives and what they really wanted. I was shocked and dismayed at how many people flouted guidance and lived their lives without a care for anyone else. After everything I'd seen and heard I couldn't hack it when people of privilege put others in danger because they claimed they were finding lockdown so difficult and so why shouldn't they break the rules. In reality, their lives had remained almost untouched by the brutalities of the situation we found ourselves in. Many hadn't lost anyone close to them and had kept their job and a roof over their heads. The sheer ignorance from some of those people about what was really going on in sectors of society was astounding and it made me so angry.

Covid has been a great amplifier of social inequality and I saw that at work in the faces of women who had been beaten up by their partners; single parents who had lost what little support network they had; people who were living with the after-effects of trauma whose safety net had been dragged out from underneath them; and countless others.

To some extent everyone was in it together and a part of something bigger, but there was a widening gulf between the haves and the have-nots in society. Being locked up in a house with a garden was not the same as being trapped in an overcrowded inner-city housing estate. Some people had lost their livelihoods and some were forced to work in dangerous conditions, while others could carry on working from the comfort of their home. Everyone was united in wanting the pandemic to end, but individual circumstances were not the same for everyone. They had never been the same.

As ever, the voices of those that needed to be heard weren't anywhere near as audible as they should have been. They were being forgotten because it was convenient.

The coronavirus pandemic had been an unimaginable disaster with more lives lost or damaged than I thought possible, but in amongst the sadness and tragedy were tales of survival and hope. It was important to remember all the positives I'd seen as well as acknowledge and work through some of the more unsavoury aspects of human nature I'd experienced. That was an ongoing and lifelong task.

Would this pandemic ever really end? Perhaps, but looking too far into the future was an impossible task. All anyone knew was that the world would never be the same again. That's the thing about endings. They are complicated. They are long and messy, full of twists and turns, a bit like the pandemic, and life itself.

Acknowledgements

From Louise:
To my sister, for reading my emotional letter and suggesting I share my story.

To Sarah, for listening to me and turning my speech into prose.

To Macmillan and Luigi, thank you for allowing me the opportunity to share my thoughts and experiences.

To my A&E family – you're the main reason I keep coming to work. And to the patients, thank you for your experiences that have given me the tales within this book. I will endeavour to do my best for you.

To Ed, for your never-ending patience, love and cooking.

Finally, to my parents for giving me a wealth of experience and always supporting me in whatever path I have chosen to follow. I love you and Dad, I miss you.

From Sarah:

I decided to write Louise's story to shine a light on the dedication of NHS staff, as well as some of the individuals in society who suffer, survive and live with terrible circumstances, and whose voices often go unheard.

I see A&E as a microcosm of society at large and a place where humanity is on display in all its forms. Within its walls, people experience emotions in extreme; there is care, chaos, beauty, destruction, compassion, love, hate, grief and so much more. I thought it would be the perfect place to set a story of how the coronavirus pandemic engulfed the country and its inhabitants, while also highlighting the deep inequality that is so rife in today's world.

I hope I've done justice to Louise, as well as her colleagues and patients. It has been a daunting and humbling task, but one that I've loved taking on.

My first thank you must go to Louise, who allowed me to tell her story and has patiently answered all my questions and laid her life bare with such honesty. When I hear about her work, I'm reassured that there are people in this world who make it a better place.

Like Louise, I'd like to thank our agent Luigi, along with Hannah, and our editor Ingrid, Alice and the wider team at Macmillan. Thanks for taking a chance on us and backing us all the way.

This book wouldn't have happened without Daniel Bunyard. Thank you for reaching out and being so kind. Your words encouraged me and gave me hope.

I worked full time reporting on the pandemic while writing this. I couldn't have done it without the steadfast love and support of my family. My friends also held me up and encouraged me when I had moments of self-doubt. Special mentions must go to Becky and Mary. Thank you to all my other friends with whom I share such great memories, and who believe in me and are there for me at different times in my life. Lexie, Katie, Sarah, Anna, Aimee, Ben, Yamine, Katherine, James, Hala, Amy, Radhika . . . there are too many to name. I'm blessed to have so many wonderful people in my life.

Massive appreciation for Emma, who read my words and provided such great thoughts and feedback. Next time, don't apologize so much!